My Journey with
Emma

A MEMOIR OF
HEALING, HOPE, & TRUTH

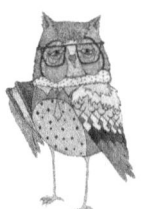

Published by
Our Written Lives of Hope, LLC

Our Written Lives of Hope provides publishing services for authors in various educational, religious, and human service organizations. For information, visit www.OurWrittenLives.com.

All rights reserved. No part of this publication may be reproduced, stored in a retrieval system, or transmitted in any form or by any means, without the permission of the copyright holder.

Copyright ©2017 Kim Houser
Cover & Interior Design by Our Written Lives

Library of Congress Cataloging-in-Publication Data
Houser, Kim 1972
My Journey with Emma: A Memoir of Healing, Hope, and Truth

Library of Congress Control Number: 2017902997
ISBN: 978-1-942923-19-0 (paperback)

Scriptures are from various Bible versions, as cited in the text.

My Journey with *Emma*

A MEMOIR OF HEALING, HOPE, & TRUTH

KIM HOUSER

Dedication

For Emma.
That your life and our journey together
may bring hope and comfort to others.

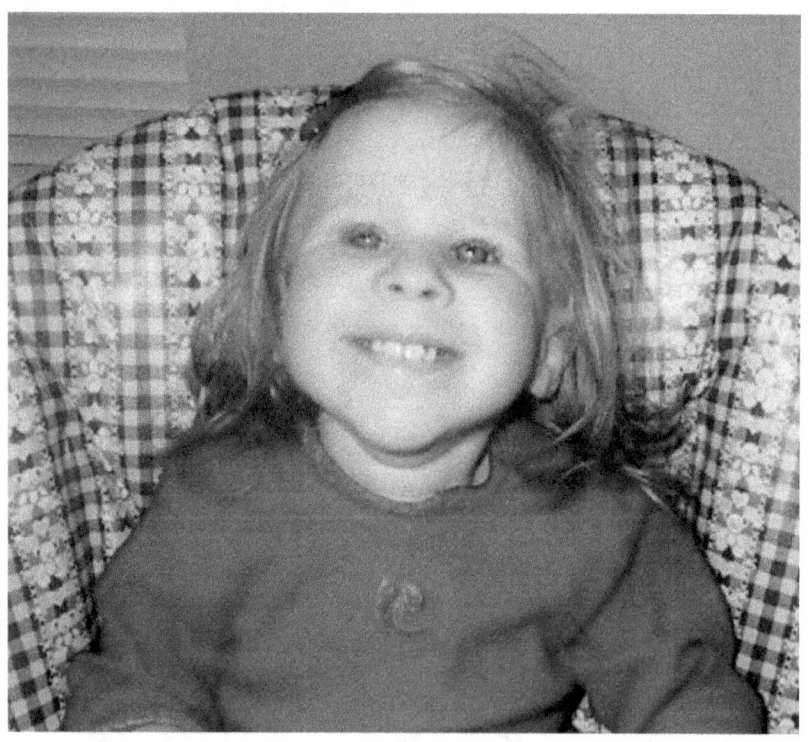

For all who face Cockayne Syndrome.
That you might relate to our story and know you are never alone.

Contents

Introduction 7
1: Truth be Told 11
2: Three Hearts 15
3: The Journey Begins 21
4: Our Tiny Enigma 27
5: Intervention & Denial 35
6: I'm Not Special 43
7: Out of the Darkness 49
8: A Wish Come True 53
9: Decline 57
10: Walking Through the Shadow 61
11: Truth from my Tiny 69
12: The Butterfly 73
13: In My Dreams 77
14: Define Normal 83
15: We Give Thanks 87
16: Too Much Reality 95
17: Lessons from my Children 101
18: Be Still and Know 105
19: Legacy 109
Acknowledgments 115
About the Author 117

My Journey with *Emma*

introduction

"Never would she be able to cling to the mercy of Heaven till she had recovered this other half which was now held fast in the deep water ... And then He gave her back her lost soul ..."
Hans Christian Andersen

Emma. The enigma child. The one born with fiery red hair.
The child who left us when she was three.
The one who now dances in heaven.

While here on earth she was always in my arms. I know I will see her again one day. My faith has grown with every stinging tear. My heart shattered, but I found peace in the midst of pain.

This is my story. It is the journey I took with my daughter Emma. It is the unraveling of myself.

Truth lies deep within each of us, yet is not always what we show to the world. Living out the truth requires a faith, which escaped me most of my life. The first thirty something years, I lived trying to make those around me believe I had everything under control.

I had an external façade I showed to the world. I didn't let others see the imperfect person I truly was. I believed life was about having a big house, spunky children, and a picture-perfect family. I wanted the world to see I had it altogether. My house was clean, insanely clean. I drove the car I thought was the best and believed staying a certain weight would bring me happiness. I found my identity in materialistic things and in believing I could control the circumstances in my life.

Despite all of this, an internal yearning to live authentically grew within me.

Then one of my children was diagnosed with a terminal illness, which I had absolutely no control over. It impacted everything I believed about *myself, my family, and my faith*. I was desperate for truth, for peace, for identity. I was desperate for God. After Emma left, my quest to live truth and find my identity in Christ became a necessary part of my healing. No longer afraid of being vulnerable, I let the walls of the façade, which I had held up for so many years, crumble around me.

I'm just me now. No façade. I'm telling my story, and revealing all my imperfections. It can be ugly at times, but my story is real and it's covered with grace. I'm fully aware pain is laced within my truth and that telling the story of my life with Emma will allow others see into the heart of an imperfect person—me. Being vulnerable and imperfect is humbling for it reveals the heart of God. I am not strong, but He is.

Realizing the truth about myself unmasked a deep faith within me. Truth gave me a clearer view of the world, and taught me where my identity actually lies. My epiphany was a result of Emma's earthly life and untimely death. Emma's life was full of purpose and I am thankful for the impact she made. I am at peace with her life and her death.

My peace is perhaps the most difficult thing for others to comprehend. How can I be completely at peace with my daughter dying? How can any mother be at peace with her child dying? Emma's death was an immensely difficult reality for me to absorb. My journey in finding joy, peace, and truth continues daily within me.

While Emma was sick, a friend said to me, "If I were you I would have already been hiding in a corner unable to face the world." For some reason, I never did hide. My life revolved around my three children, one who had multiple special needs and a terminal illness. I always knew she would die before me, but I had to live, keep laughing, and find joy even with the knowledge that she would not be with me forever. I had to find the one true source of joy.

My journey with Emma led me through a grief process before I came to joy. I experienced denial, darkness, an unquenchable desire to make Emma healthy. Finally I accepted her disease and surrendered her physical body to the Lord.

After Emma passed away, my son Peyton begged to see the movie *Cars*. I read an excerpt from the movie and discovered there was a lesson to be learned from its story line. The lesson was that life is more about enjoying the journey than winning the race. Though there has been much pain, my journey has brought me much joy. Ultimately, it has been a quest for my own healing.

The person I was before Emma was born no longer exists. All my past conceptions of what a fulfilled life looked like are now torn apart. What is left is an ever-ripening wisdom that living life is not to be defined by others' expectations. A fulfilled life is not measured by accomplishments, wealth, or the amount of time we spend on earth. The brief flickering of time that was Emma's life held more meaning and fullness than many people ever experience. I now know life is about the journey we take with one another, and our relationship with God. I know that every long, solitude, stretch of highway, and each unpredictable hairpin curve is part of our growth. Life is not the ending, but the journey itself, which teaches us truth.

I don't feel brave or heroic because I survived the death of one of my children. Instead, I am humbled by the lessons I learned after my old reality shattered. The brokenness began with Emma's diagnosis at age two. It was a rare illness called Cockayne Syndrome, a recessively inherited genetic disorder, which causes rapid aging symptoms. Emma

My Journey with Emma

had Cockayne Syndrome Type 2, which usually results in the child passing away before the age of seven.

We called her our "Little Bit." Emma was strong, courageous, tiny and full of spunk. She was never able to speak, but Emma and I had our own language, our own deep connection. I completely understood her as I looked through her eyes and saw right into her soul. Her existence gave me strength, and I found hope reflected in her eyes. She taught me every day like a spring-fed well of truth. But the lessons Emma's life brought didn't come easy to me. Denial and anger about her diagnosis haunted me for a very long time before I found hope.

Hope filled my soul as my faith grew. At times, my faith was so strong I felt as if God literally lifted and carried me through the pain. But the pain of saying goodbye to her was very real and seared me emotionally. Trusting God has been the greatest struggle of all, but it was the only way I could balance the crushing pain with hope. I learned that if I were to find hope and truth, I must relinquish all power to God.

It is my hope that as I share the depths of my pain along with the boundless joy I discovered, that I may help others find their truth and a glimpse of hope along the journey. At times my story is heartbreaking and raw. I began writing during Emma's life and continued after she died.

You will read of *My Journey with Emma*, from the time of her birth, through the pain of saying goodbye to her, and what came after. I have learned to embrace pain along my quest for truth. Inexplicably, pain and grace intertwine to bring us to the most important truth God has for us. We grow through pain, but we do not have to stay in the suffering. May any facades you carry fall away as you journey with me.

Truth be Told

chapter one

"Hear my cry, O God; attend to my prayer." Psalm 61:1

From My Journal - December 2004
I fake my strength sometimes. My facade is making me crazy. If I could scream out the truth maybe the panicked filled days would be calm.

My soul began to sink into a primal dark abyss of fear inside of me. Waves of nausea swept over me as the front door closed with a resounding thud. The house had grown silent, but as I turned away from the door my thoughts began exploding like fireworks.

"How can it already be time for this? We haven't had her long enough! This isn't really happening!"

Each thought felt like tiny shreds of glass piercing through my skin. Truth swelled my heart with a bitter, stinging pain. My mind was crazy with reality as my body filled with overwhelming emotion.

Two women from hospice had just left my home. One was a tall, protective woman with glasses—a social worker. The other was short and stodgy, a clinical nurse with great knowledge of aging and its symptoms. They had listened to my litany of concerns as we sat in my living room. An icy level of tension hung in the air while they evaluated my daughter Emma's health and gave me their recommendations.

"She appears to be showing signs of pre-mature aging," the nurse said. Emma's face was gaunt, with dark circles under her eyes. The women watched as Emma began throwing up the entire contents of her stomach, everything she had eaten the previous night.

"That is a sign her stomach is slowing down. It happens when people get much older," the nurse said with both concern and perplexity.

Emma seemed to resemble a ninety-year-old woman rather than a three-year-old child. She was losing her eyesight and her breathing was shallow. Both women felt she was ready for hospice based on her symptoms and the crude timeline for children living with Cockayne Syndrome. They advised me to contact her pediatrician as soon as possible to get approval for Emma's admittance into hospice care.

The women politely said goodbye, and I briefly marked their exit by staring at their figures through the front windows as they solemnly walked down the long, brick walkway to the car. I had worked in social services for years and knew they were masking their emotion while in our home. I knew it was bad. Emma was very, very sick. I collapsed onto the carpeted stairs across from our front door and struggled to breathe.

My façade of smiles and ease in handling the meeting with the women masked an internal fear, which now threatened to overtake my grip on saneness. Not many knew about my severe panic attacks. Now, in the wake of this meeting, my body began to hyperventilate as I gasped for air, and tried to stop wild panic from consuming my mind. Heaving sobs came from my exhausted body, but I stifled them trying not to wake the two children who were napping just a few feet from me.

Paige, my one-year-old, slumbered peacefully in her baby bed after the kind of active morning most toddlers have. Through the door of the other bedroom, I could hear the motor of the feeding machine clicking as it pumped liquid food into my tiny three-year-old daughter Emma's tummy. We had to continue keeping her hydrated with small amounts of liquid, even though she had thrown up earlier. She had fallen asleep moments before in the pretty, lavender colored room

Chapter 1 — Truth be Told

with butterflies hanging from the ceiling, totally unaware she was the focus of the hospice meeting.

A week earlier, in a huge sigh of courage, I had requested an in-home evaluation from a hospice organization. My husband and I needed to know if it was time. Was our daughter Emma in the last stage of her terminal illness? She had just turned three a mere five months earlier.

I breathed in deeply, exhaled fear, and pulled myself together as I prepared to pick up my four-year-old son Peyton from preschool. Why had I insisted on having the meeting with hospice alone? Why did I always try to do everything by myself, refusing to ask for help?

After the two social workers left my home, reality sunk in. I must start asking for and accepting help from others. This meeting confirmed my darkest suspicion. *Emma was dying and I had to stop trying to show the world a facade of strength.*

I painted a Van Gogh of capability, a face full of makeup and smiles, and kept everyone at arms length from the truth that I was falling apart on the inside. Like a master illusionist, I created a vision of strength. My friends told me I was strong, and they wouldn't be able to handle my circumstances if they were in my shoes. But that morning I felt defeated, alone, and more scared than I had ever felt in my life.

Truth was ripping apart the illusion. Reality and truth were crashing into my world and I had to face each one head on, knowing it would be a struggle to keep myself, my marriage, my family, and my friendships intact. I always had faith God existed, but now I must begin relinquishing control, and finding strength in Him.

The sun loomed on the horizon, and it was time to take off all my masks. It was the only way I could fully absorb the peace and hope that comes from resting in God's presence along the journey. That morning, as I sat on the stairs feeling helpless, images of my life before Emma was born began to fill my mind.

Three Hearts

chapter two

"The smallest of them will become a family. The weakest of them will become a mighty nation. At the right time I, the LORD, will make it happen quickly." Isaiah 60:22

Peyton heard the truck pulling into the driveway, looked at me with a grin, and mumbled, "Da Da?"

Scooping him up, I said, "Yes, Peyton bug! Your daddy is home."

As Eli walked in the house, six-month-old Peyton reached for him saying, "Da Da! Da Da!" over and over again until my husband took him from my arms.

"Hey, big guy! Hey, Goose!" Eli said to us both. Goose was the nickname Eli had called me since we met at age nineteen.

Evenings were always a fun time for our family of three. From the moment Eli came home Peyton begged for his attention. We were married six years before having a child and Peyton was the center of our lives.

Eli owned a landscaping company, which did well enough financially to allow me to stay home with Peyton. I spent my days making sure Peyton's life was full of happiness, love, and attention. We spent hours playing silly games and reading books.

As a first-time mom I was very unsure of my capabilities and read all sorts of books advising me on raising a well-rounded, well-behaved child. I wanted to be a great mom, but what I didn't realize was that perfect parenting doesn't exist. Thankfully, grace is so much more powerful than our expectations.

My Journey with *Emma*

Through my days alone with Peyton, I began to realize how much I really wanted to bond with other moms. I wanted to share stories of sleepless nights, shirts soaked in spit-up, loads of laundry that seemed to breed, and how taking a shower had suddenly become a luxury. Finding a "mom friend" was harder than I thought.

We were invited to a playgroup when Peyton was six months old. I eagerly accepted, looking forward to meeting the other moms. I arrived right on time and rang the doorbell. When the mom who hosted the playgroup opened the door, I wondered if Peyton and I were in the right place.

She had on a belt.

There is nothing wrong with wearing belts, but at that time, I didn't even wear my shirts tucked in—not after having a baby. It took entirely too much time to look pulled together enough to wear a belt. I could barely make it out of the house with a shower.

Seeing the belted-mother I sighed internally and thought, *"Will anyone here even have spit-up on their clothes?"* I wasn't so sure.

Soft, melodic music flowed throughout her home. The house was immaculate and her son was in a plaid, baby-blue outfit that had his name embroidered on the front.

Peyton had on a jumper with a dump truck on it that said, "Dig."

I had Birkenstock's on my feet, my shirt was not tucked in, and I didn't even own a belt.

But it was a play date where other adults would be present, and I needed friends. I took a deep breath and told myself it would be okay.

As the other moms arrived, I realized it might not be okay. All the other moms at the group were more interested in discussing where they had purchased their children's embroidered, monogrammed clothing, or where the host had acquired her fine china—which we were using for our snacks.

CHAPTER 2 *Three Hearts*

Buckling Peyton into his car seat after the two-hour play-date disaster, I whispered, "It's okay, buddy. I like your dump truck outfit. We will find some friends for us, I promise!"

"Da Da?" He said looking at me with wide, green, soulful eyes.

"Good grief, will this child ever say Mama?" I thought.

A few weeks later while grocery shopping, I met a young mom with a little girl who looked to be around Peyton's age. We were both standing on the baby aisle peering at jars of food. She smiled at me and asked how old Peyton was.

We began talking and had a lot in common. Our children were the same age, she mentioned being sleep deprived, and I thought I noticed a tiny bit of strained bananas on the back of her shirt. Things looked promising. Peyton and Riley grinned shyly at one another as Amy and I exchanged phone numbers.

We formed a fast friendship. We spent hours at one another's homes watching the kids play, chatting about our childhood, marriage, and raising our children. Amy was easygoing and fun to be around. For the most part, Riley and Peyton got along, but there were a few biting incidents. Neither child had a sibling, so they were learning the not-so-fine art of sharing and taking turns. At least that is what Amy and I hoped was happening. We were all just happy to have company. She hadn't made any "mommy friends" either, since having Riley.

Sometimes our conversation would turn toward our thoughts on having more children. Amy wanted at least one more. I knew I wanted many children, but didn't know if that would ever be a reality. Eli and I were still trying to get down the art of parenting one child.

A few months after I met Amy, the weather turned cooler and I started feeling odd. I was constantly starving, and felt bloated. One morning, I tossed a bag of old Halloween candy at Eli and yelled, "Take this to work! I can't stop eating it!" He laughed, but took the candy to keep me from going on a tirade about how fat I was feeling.

After he left, I picked up the phone and called my OB-GYN to schedule a checkup. When the secretary asked why, I replied, "Because I feel bloated, I am crying all the time, and I can't stop eating chocolate. I think I need a pregnancy test."

As I sat in the doctor's office waiting on the results of the test, I looked over at Peyton who was sitting in his stroller staring at a self-breast exam chart hanging on the wall.

"How in the world could I possibly be pregnant?" I asked out loud to the empty room. It had taken years to have Peyton. We didn't think we would ever have children. We were going through infertility testing when we found out I was pregnant the first time. Eli and I had always wanted more children, but we felt Peyton might be our only child. We were content with our family of three and didn't imagine God was going to expand our number to four any time soon.

Dr. Bishop came into the room with a huge grin on her face. "Guess what? You're pregnant!" She said with excitement.

"What? Are you sure?" I asked as butterflies of excitement danced in my stomach.

"Yes, your due date is July 13th," she replied.

I wondered if Eli was going to be as happy as I was to hear the news. Driving through the parking garage, I dialed him on my cell phone.

"Guess what, Honey?" I asked.

"What?"

"I'm pregnant!"

"Huh?"

"We are having a baby! I'm due in July!"

Silence.

In hindsight, I suppose it was a bit of a shocker to tell him over the phone. When he got home that evening he still seemed dazed. I hugged him and asked how he was feeling.

Chapter 2 — Three Hearts

"I'm nervous about having them so close together, about being able to financially support two children in diapers," he said. By the time the new baby was born, our kids would be only eighteen months apart.

I assured Eli it would be okay and that we would get through it just like we got through everything—together. He still seemed scared, but I went to bed with dreams of watching two children peering out the front door saying "Daddy" as they waited on my husband to get home from work. In my dream there was a little girl standing beside Peyton. Her head was covered in red curls.

About two months into my pregnancy Amy and I took the kids to Chick-Fil-A for an outing lunch and she beamed as she blurted out her news. "I'm pregnant!"

"AWE! I am so excited for you!" I screamed. I think everyone in Chick-Fil-A heard me.

Our conversation turned to the future. The following summer there would be four little ones to fill our days. We talked about taking all four kids to the park, and watching them fight over toys. It was so good to have a friend who was at the same stage in life as me. Our pregnancies progressed and all seemed well with each of us.

Eli and I decided not to find out if we were having a boy or a girl. When my step-mother painted the nursery a beautiful lavender color, Eli jokingly commented, "A boy can't sleep in that room. We will have to re-paint it if this baby is a boy," he said.

My dreams kept telling me we wouldn't have to re-paint the room. I was so excited about having another baby, but I worried about Peyton not getting enough attention. He was our entire world for the past eighteen months. How was I going to love another child as much as I loved my green-eyed boy?

The Journey Begins

chapter three

*"You formed my inmost being; you knit me in my mother's womb ...
Your eyes foresaw my actions; in your book all are written down; my
days were shaped, before one came to be."*
Psalms 139:13, 16

Before she was born, we already decided if the baby was a girl we'd call her Emma. The name "Emma" lingered in my mind throughout my pregnancy. Somehow it seemed no other name would fit the soul living within me. Eli wasn't fond of the name, and we fiercely debated until one week before her birth when he finally conceded and said, "I kind of like the name now." And so it was decided. Our unborn child became Emma.

We didn't know the meaning of her name when we decided on it. She was two years old before we researched the meaning, and it was a long while after that before I began to realize how perfectly her name fit her sweet spirit. Emma means "one who heals."

We chose her middle name, Catherine, after my grandmother. My grandmother Catherine had many grandchildren and great grandchildren but none had ever been named after her. When I was sixteen years old I was very close to her and listened to her lament that another great-grandchild had been born in the family and the baby hadn't been named after her. I always loved my grandmother's name and promised her that if I ever had a little girl I would name her Catherine. My grandmother was elated when Emma was born and we named her Emma Catherine. I loved the name Catherine because it means "pure."

Emma was born on a hot summer morning, July 6, 2001. The hospital room bustled with doctors, nurses and excitement. Because Peyton had been born via c-section and Emma was born only a year and a half after his birth, my doctor recommended another C-Section.

Eli and I went to the hospital early that Friday morning and prepared to welcome our newest child. Emma's birth was a much easier experience than Peyton's, who had taken 24 hours to finally enter the world. With Emma, I was calm and relaxed.

Emma's birth brought heightened anticipation and excitement because we didn't know whether we were having a girl or a boy. Through the window of the sterile hospital room, I could see a magnificent backdrop. The rising sun filled the sky with deep hues of indigo and crimson. It seemed to mirror the warmth in my heart.

I was prepped for surgery and Eli put on scrubs to be in the room with me. We held hands as the doctor and nurses began the C-Section. I couldn't wait to find out if Peyton would have a little sister, or brother. In what seemed an instant, we had a little girl.

Her newborn cry pierced the room with its pitch and fury. They handed Emma to me and my journey with this amazing child began.

Eli and I inhaled joy, exhaled relief, and gazed with wonder upon the tiny face of our second child, Emma Catherine.

We fell in love with her immediately. She was bundled in a scratchy hospital receiving blanket, and only her tiny, crimson red face peeked out.

I remember that sunny July morning as I held her, I looked at her with a mix of pride and something incomprehensible. Was it fear? As I peered at her with curiosity, a strange thought consumed me.

"What is wrong with my child?" I wondered silently.

CHAPTER 3 *The Journey Begins*

I kept that unspoken question locked away in the recesses of my mind. The suspicions I had on the day of her birth told me something was very wrong with Emma, yet my fears were too strong and frightening for me to utter them aloud.

I told no one, not even Eli, about the strange thoughts I had. Emma was tiny; she only weighed five pounds and ten ounces, yet she appeared healthy.

Because she was so tiny, the doctors assumed our dates were off, and that she was born a few weeks early. I pushed aside my thoughts that something was wrong with Emma.

She was so tiny that she fit into preemie clothing. Everyone was excited to have a girl in the family. She was the first granddaughter for both sides of our family and the first girl born in Eli's family in forty-two years.

Emma was a special little girl. Everyone hurried to buy gifts for her. My mom bought her a tiny pink outfit to wear for her baby photos. Even with preemie clothing, Emma looked as if she were being swallowed in all of the material. I had never held a baby so tiny. I stared into her small face and felt as if I were holding a gift from God.

While in the hospital after her birth, Emma had a lot of difficulty eating. She would cry and throw up after attempting to drink a few ounces of milk. We suspected she had reflux as Peyton did when he was born, or maybe it was even worse, something like pyloric stenosis. Peyton also had pyloric stenosis, a condition, which causes the intestine to constrict, leading to the inability to digest food, as well as severe dehydration.

If Emma had pyloric stenosis she would require surgery. Doctors began to monitor Emma for these conditions, but after two days they insisted Emma's feeding issues were related to her being an early baby, not pyloric stenosis or anything more serious. I was ready to go home and see Peyton, so we agreed with the doctors that perhaps she had been born a few weeks early. The doctors didn't feel she needed any further testing or monitoring in the hospital.

With our second child, we weren't dealing with the nerves of being new parents. Instead, we were looking forward to life with our bigger family. Although I was having odd feelings, I was still a young mom and knew all babies would bring different challenges.

Thankfully, the lavender room my stepmother painted was the perfect color. It made a sweet nursery for my baby girl. We placed a cream-colored glider rocker in the corner near a window. That quiet corner of her room became a place I would spend many hours nestling baby Emma, praying and rocking.

I was overly prepared for bringing a new baby home. Meals were stocked in the freezer and help was scheduled to come in for our first few days home.

When we introduced Peyton to Emma he was so excited. He was only a year and a half old, but was a precocious child. He called Emma "baby" and wanted to hold her and kiss her. He would stand on his tippy toes to peer down into her little bassinet, which sat in the den. He loved her. He wanted her to "get big" and "play" with him. Peyton didn't seem to act as if anything had changed in his world. It was as if Peyton had been waiting on Emma his whole life.

Once, shortly after her birth, I placed Emma in her swing, set the speed to low and sped to the bathroom. When I came out moments later, Emma was swinging rapidly, with the swing on high! Peyton was standing next to her grinning. He squealed, "Baby Emma go high!"

Peyton had turned up the swing and watched with glee as she rocked back and forth. He loved to swing high, and I suppose he thought Emma would like it too. Watching Peyton with his little sister, I knew life was going to be very busy. I had two children under

Chapter 3: The Journey Begins

the age of two and my newborn wasn't acting like a typical child. Still, we were a happy little family and we looked forward to Emma and Peyton playing together some day. Eli would come home every day and jump right in to help with the children. He would take Peyton and give him a bath, play games with him, read to him and put him to bed.

Emma was still not eating or sleeping well. I prayed she was just a difficult baby to soothe and that it was simply a matter of time before things improved. I fell asleep on the couch each night with Emma lying on my chest. This was the only way she would calm. Eventually, I moved back to the bedroom, but I had to keep Emma with me because she couldn't fall asleep unless someone was holding her upright.

While it wasn't ideal to fall asleep with a baby cradled on your chest every night, it was in these moments I felt a deep connection to my new daughter and blessed beyond measure. Eli and I weren't sure we would ever have children, and now we had two. I gazed at Emma while she was sleeping and marveled at how God brought two children into our lives in such a short amount of time.

From the very beginning of her life, Emma was a child who taught us to trust in God and to fully rely on Him for guidance. While we didn't know the gravity of Emma's condition at the time of her birth, we knew God created Emma and He would help us navigate any challenge we faced with her.

Peyton and Emma

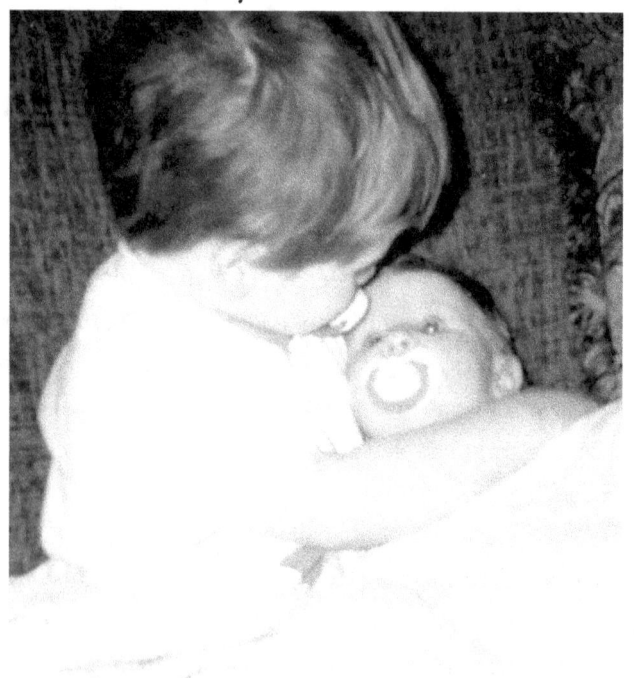

Our Tiny Enigma

chapter four

"I will always have the wonderful story of how your family has taught me more about the power of God's love and how one little girl can show you the things that are important in life."
—card from a family friend to Emma

Just like in my dreams, Emma had a head of curly red hair. No one else in our family had red hair. She was a little mystery.

Unfortunately, Emma didn't grow out of her eating problems. When she ate, she would scream as if she were in pain. She would spit-up nearly one hundred times every day. I had a bib to match every outfit she had. I would coordinate bibs for the outfits and change them daily as she threw up over and over.

Because of her issues, I took Emma to the doctor once or twice a week. I would walk into the office and politely ask what could be wrong with my baby. Her pediatrician kept telling me Emma was born four or five weeks early and was acting typical for a baby born prematurely.

Eli and I felt horrible about Emma's sickness. I thought I was to blame. I was so distracted as a new mom. I blamed myself, thinking I had given the wrong dates to my obstetrician. Maybe the C-Section was scheduled early due to my miscalculations.

The weekly visits to the doctor continued and I always received the same answer, "Remember, she was an early baby. She will grow out of the spitting up."

But what about all the screaming as if she is in pain? I wondered.

After speaking to a friend who had a little boy with severe acid reflux, I marched into the pediatrician's office and demanded Emma have a referral to a gastroenterologist to have a barium swallow done. A barium swallow would tell us if Emma had acid reflux. The look on Emma's doctor's face dared me to question her medical knowledge.

"Why do you think she has reflux?" She asked smugly.

It was evident I had been too passive in my numerous previous visits to the pediatrician. Steadfast and stern, I voiced my demand again. "Get Emma a gastroenterologist referral now!"

Grudgingly, the doctor made the call and got us an appointment. The tests showed Emma had severe acid reflux and needed three kinds of medication to repair her tiny body and help soothe the pain. Her throat was raw from weeks of acid corroding its lining. Her screams were not the cries of a fussy early baby, but from a baby in pain. Finally, I listened to my instincts and stood up to the doctor.

Eli and I had other concerns in addition to Emma constantly spitting up. She rarely opened her eyes, and when she did she would start screaming again. Her head was so tiny, only the size of a large orange. It seemed trivial at the time, but I really wanted to put one of those cute, frilly sun hats on her, and couldn't because her head was so small.

At her four-month check-up, the doctor asked me the routine questions and gave Emma a thumbs up, saying, "See you in two months." As she walked out of the door, I literally pulled the pediatrician back into the exam room and asked her emphatically, "Don't you think her head is too small?"

She examined Emma more closely, and after a few moments said, "Maybe we should get a CAT scan of her head."

I didn't know it at the time, but the doctor had written the word "microcephaly" in Emma's medical chart. I didn't know what it

CHAPTER 4 *Our Tiny Enigma*

meant anyway; I barely knew what a CAT scan was. We later learned microcephaly meant Emma's brain was not growing. Lots of problems could cause microcephaly, but the doctor's first explanation was a fixable medical problem.

She told me Emma's skull was most likely unusually small because of a medical condition called "craniosynostosis." She said maybe Emma had that huge-preposterous-diagnosis I couldn't pronounce, and might need surgery on her skull to correct the problem. My world spun inward and I cocked my head to the side as I repeated her words.

"Surgery on Emma's head?"

Nonchalantly, she replied, "Yeah! It's no big deal. We will get the CAT scan and see what it says."

I was not emotionally equipped to deal with the thought of head surgery, or anything that close to the brain, and Emma in the same sentence. But the doctor sounded so unconcerned. I thought, *"OK we can deal with this."*

I wrapped my mind around the thought of surgery for my tiny Emma. Maybe it would fix whatever problem had been lurking unspoken since the inception of her life. My mind began to plan.

"We can fix this problem. We will have to get the best referrals, doctors, and opinions."

After the doctor ordered the test, she continued to assure me Emma would develop just fine and at her own pace. Still, I had a haunting feeling that something was very wrong with my daughter.

The CAT scan showed Emma's brain development was normal. She did not have craniosynostosis. The news was a huge relief and my extended family members told me to quit worrying about Emma. She was just "little," they said. She would grow at her own pace.

Early one morning, a week after her CAT scan and the "normal" diagnosis, Emma began having seizures and violent vomiting. Her eyes rolled back into her head, her body began to shake with tremors for nearly two hours, and I thought she was dying.

Peyton slept upstairs in his room as I frantically called Eli, my mom, and every doctor Emma had at that time. I had to find help. One doctor said, "I know it is hard to watch when they shake while throwing up from reflux." Thankfully, my mom took time off work and hurried over to the house to help out.

Instinct told me this horrid experience pointed to something more serious than reflux or the "early baby symptoms" everyone had drilled into my mind for four months. I rushed Emma to the doctor and stood by as they drew her blood. The blood work indicated Emma had a bacterial infection. The doctor gave her a high dose injection of antibiotics and told me to bring her in the next day to make sure her antibodies had lowered.

Inside the exam room the next day, the doctor sat me down and with a look of trepidation on her face she said, "You need to take Emma to the ER. Her blood tests today are showing even higher levels of antibodies indicating she is fighting something much worse than we thought. My hunch is childhood cancer."

Strapping Emma into her car seat, I drove in a trance-like state to the hospital. Along the way I called my mom to meet me. I also called to make sure my babysitter could stay longer with Peyton. It was going to be a long time before either Eli or I could return home.

Life was morphing into something worse than I could imagine. While pathologists looked at Emma's blood under microscopes, I sat in shock in an ER hospital room watching nurses prick and poke at Emma in order to have multiple blood tests and exams completed.

Emma was so tiny. She didn't even weigh twelve pounds, even though she was four months old. All she wanted was for me to hold her. Just take her home and hold her. It's what I wanted too. For the

CHAPTER 4 Our Tiny Enigma

past four months she had slept on my chest, our two hearts almost beating as one. She would cry from the pain of the reflux, soothed only when she was nestled up against my neck. Her entire body was only the length of a dishtowel.

The tests showed Emma did not have childhood cancer, but she was admitted to the hospital and started on high doses of IV antibiotics anyway. Obviously, her body was fighting some kind of infection. The doctors continued to run tests and give her medications, but her white count crept higher and higher. Still suspecting childhood cancer, the doctors transferred Emma to Children's of Alabama, the pediatric hospital in Birmingham. Emma was admitted around midnight.

Eli and I were exhausted mentally and physically as we began another round of watching Emma go through more tests and blood work. The doctors asked me if Eli and I were related. We were exhausted, and probably looked horrible on the outside, but both of us giggled as they asked if we were related. At the time we thought they were judging us by how we appeared. We didn't realize they suspected Emma might have a genetic illness.

Infectious disease specialists were called in and I was tested for possible maternal infections that could have been passed on to Emma during my pregnancy. Every single test came back normal. After one week, her white count mysteriously dropped and the doctors were stumped. One of the doctors mentioned Emma may have some form of dwarfism, but felt that was just a symptom of a larger problem.

My mom and I sat in the hospital room tears rolling down both of our faces.

"Do you think she will ever be able to walk?" My mom asked as she rocked Emma.

"We just don't know right now what is going on, or what her future will be like," the doctor answered.

We had so many questions, but no one had any answers. After nearly two weeks of tests and spending our Thanksgiving eating in the hospital cafeteria, Emma was discharged. We packed our things and went home, utterly confused.

The doctors were positive about one thing. They didn't know Emma's full diagnosis, but they assured us she was not an "early baby," as her pediatrician had suggested for the past four months. She did have microcephaly of unknown origin. It was one piece to the puzzle that would eventually unravel her full diagnosis.

The doctors told us to keep a list of her many symptoms, and to watch her growth progress. I knew they suspected something, but only time would reveal the truth. I also knew I would continue searching for an answer. Emma was my little girl and I wanted more than anything to see her standing beside her brother at the front door, waiting for Eli to walk in the door.

We would find what was wrong. We would fix Emma. We had to. I still believed I was in control.

As Eli and I were leaving Birmingham that last day, we entered an elevator with two women and a child in a wheelchair. The child was completely covered with a hat, glasses, and a blanket over his body. It was obvious the sun was harmful to him. I thought to myself, "*He is one of those children who can't be in the sun.*" I couldn't remember the name of the disease. The women with him seemed strong, and so equipped to deal with the stares and special measures to keep a single of ray of sun from hitting this special child's skin.

Over the past four months, truth whispered deep into my subconscious, sending me subtle clues about Emma's condition. Looking back, the first clue I had was when Emma was around eight weeks old. She had a blistering sunburn after being outside in the shade for only ten minutes.

CHAPTER 4 *Our Tiny Enigma*

The pediatrician insisted we had exposed her to chemicals from pesticides Eli sometimes worked with, which had likely caused the severe burn on her face. Knowing we had not done anything to harm Emma, I pleaded with the doctor to find an answer for Emma's sunburn.

"Doesn't it look more like a sunburn to you?" I asked her pediatrician.

"No, it is too severe to be a sunburn," she replied.

As I sat in the room with Emma I could hear nurses whispering outside the closed door. I was numb and scared from what I heard them saying.

"Did you see that baby's face? What did they do to her?" They mumbled.

I fully believed they were going to call Child Protective Services on our family, but I knew we had done nothing to put our child in harm's way.

Most concerning was the fact that I felt none of the doctors or nurses listened to me. I knew the odd rash and burn was caused by the sun, and not from chemicals. Emma had to take antibiotics for the burn and I put a special cream on her scaling face for weeks until it healed. We took extra precautions by placing sun blockers on our car windows where Emma was exposed. We kept Emma out of the sunlight as much as possible.

I started doing my own research on the internet, searching for the answer to my daughter's medical problems. Typing in microcephaly, sunburn, dwarfism, and reflux, I found horrible syndromes. The growing list of symptoms was linked to something deeper, and like a puzzle, the pieces slowly began to come together.

I felt as if I were racing against time as I spent hours researching rare illnesses, negative reactions to vaccinations, and even the possibility of tainted drinking water in our area.

As I searched for answers, I knew Emma met the criteria for several syndromes. Each syndrome always had "shortened life expectancy" on the list of symptoms. Those three words fueled me to continue searching for another answer. Shortened life expectancy was something I could *not* accept.

I found myself feeling deep sadness over my perceived "loss" of a typical child and found it difficult to even spend time with my friend Amy, whose son was close in age to Emma. I was very happy for my friends with typical children but deeply afraid of what the future may hold for Emma.

A close family member told me I had become too absorbed with Emma. She said I was obsessed with taking care of her increasing special needs, and seeking answers to her undiagnosed condition. Incensed by her words, I worked even harder to find answers and help for Emma.

One of the most important lessons Eli and I had to learn about being the parents of a child with special needs was that we were her primary voice, the main advocates. My character is submissive, usually afraid to speak up or make people angry. I always had a need to be liked, so I usually kept my opinions to myself. Learning how to stand up to doctors was an intimidating task, but something I was slowly learning to do.

Over time, my husband and I learned we knew what our child needed even more than the doctors did. We both were previously conditioned to believe doctors knew everything. We put so much trust into the doctor's capabilities, but when it came to Emma we had to rely on what we knew about her instead of what the doctor's textbooks told them about our daughter.

Intervention & Denial

chapter five

From My Journal
You speak no words but say so much to every heart that listens to you.
Some are frightened of you because of your outward special needs,
but those who believe see God in your eyes, and in your spirit.
Sometimes, I think you are the bravest of us all.

When Emma turned eight months old, her primary diagnosis was still "Microcephaly of Unknown Origin." I struggled emotionally with the lack of clear answers. An evaluation by United Cerebral Palsy (UCP) said Emma met the criteria for early intervention and showed a significant delay in developmental and physical skills. She began early intervention services when she was seven months old. UCP provided physical therapy, speech therapy, and occupational therapy.

I learned of a support group through UCP, which could help me connect with other moms who understood what it was like to have a child with special needs. I began attending a meeting called "Moms to Special Children."

A few moments after I sat down at the first meeting, a lady walked in and sat next to me. She had no children with her and I soon realized she was the guest speaker that night.

She began asking me questions about Emma, who was sitting in her car seat cooing and looking around at everyone with interest. The lady was enamored with Emma and wanted to hold her. Each question she asked was eerily right on target with every symptom Emma had.

"Does she have tight joints? Does she have reflux? Microcephaly?"

"Yes. Yes." I repeated after every single question.

"Who was this lady? Was she a doctor, or a nurse? And why does she know to ask all these questions?" I wondered silently.

The woman exhaled and asked, "Does she sunburn easily?"

My eyes widened. "Yes, even in the shade," I quietly replied.

She slammed her hand onto the table and said with certainty and a level of shock in her voice, "She has Cockayne Syndrome!"

The woman whipped out a photo of her little girl, Hannah, who amazingly looked very similar to Emma. Then she spoke words I will never forget.

"This is my Hannah. She had Cockayne Syndrome," the woman said.

Zoning in on the word "had," I didn't want to hear the next words out of her mouth.

"Hannah passed away two years ago at age four and half, but she had a very rare form of the syndrome." The woman gave me the names of doctors to contact. I could tell she didn't want to frighten me, but she knew too much about my daughter and I had an odd feeling our meeting was the result of divine intervention.

It was that very moment, in the middle of an encounter with a complete stranger, when I began to build an invisible wall around myself. It was a wall of denial to protect me from the painful truth. Still, nothing could stop the subtle voice, which had whispered to me for eight months, from breathing truth into my universe.

Emma will die before me.

The question that haunted me on the day of Emma's birth finally had an answer. Something in me knew I would never again ask the question, "What is wrong with my child?"

Immediately after I left the support group, I called Emma's pediatric neurologist, Dr. Teasley. She was an astounding doctor we began

CHAPTER 5 *Intervention & Denial*

seeing when Emma was four months old, just after our stay at the Children's Hospital of Birmingham.

On the phone with the nurse, I sputtered out the name Cockayne Syndrome. The nurse she said she would call me back after speaking to the doctor.

Dr. Teasley had extensive experience with children who had rare syndromes. She had a remarkable reputation, and a lot of quirks. She would carry her large gray purse into every child's appointment. Every time she walked into the exam room, she would drop her overstuffed purse onto the exam table, never acknowledging its presence. I was always acutely aware and curious about that purse. It wasn't a medical bag with exam equipment. From all observations, it was simply her purse. I later learned she was known in the special needs community as, "Dr. Teasley: teeming full of great knowledge, and owner of the enormous purse of mystery."

Despite her oddities, she was attentive, patient, and genuinely enjoyed learning how to best care for Emma's health. These were qualities Emma's first pediatrician never displayed.

The nurse called me back later that day and said, "Dr. Teasley doesn't think it could be Cockayne Syndrome. Cockayne is so rare there isn't even a test for it."

Still, the doctor ordered MRI scans just to provide additional medical knowledge of what may be happening. The results came back normal—another test and another normal conclusion. Children with Cockayne Syndrome were supposed to have brain changes and problems evident in MRI's. Emma didn't have those problems according to the MRI.

A few months later I took Emma 500 miles away to a renowned children's neurologist in Houston, Texas. He walked in the room, looked at Emma for about ten minutes, and in a thick Australian accent said, "Cockayne Syndrome." I had never mentioned my suspicion about Cockayne to him. He told me he had seen children like her, and he was very sorry, but he knew what he was talking about.

I left his office shaking. As I carried ten-month-old Emma in my arms, it felt as if my whole world was ending. Now a medical doctor had breathed those words into the air, "Cockayne Syndrome."

Trying to think rationally, Eli and I focused on the statistics for occurrences of Cockayne. There couldn't possibly be two cases in the same city. Anne, the lady I had met at the Moms to Special Children meeting two months earlier, also lived in our city. Cockayne Syndrome was only supposed to happen in one out of every 500,000 births. Our city was not that large.

After bringing Emma back home to Alabama, I met with her neurologist, Dr. Teasley and discussed Cockayne Syndrome with her again. She knew and respected the doctor I had seen in Texas and agreed to look at Emma's MRI scans once more. She and her business partner, another child neurologist, both concluded that the MRI scans were normal. The doctor in Houston vehemently disagreed and said there were mild abnormalities in Emma's scan, the type of problems seen in children with Cockayne Syndrome.

Still searching for answers, I found out there was one lab in the United States that could test for Cockayne Syndrome and we began to prepare to have Emma's skin biopsy done. Fate stepped in again, slamming the breaks on finding a sure answer. Sadly, the only Cockayne expert who offered testing in the United States had died suddenly. Emma's questionable diagnosis hung over our heads like a thick, black cloud.

The only firm diagnosis at that time was microcephaly and developmental delay. The doctor recommended another expert, one on genetic microcephaly, and we sent Emma's MRI scans to Chicago.

CHAPTER 5 *Intervention & Denial*

That doctor also said the scans looked normal, but confirmed Emma did have microcephaly of unknown origin. Countless doctors, specialists and tests, and they all said something different. Unsure of which specialist was correct, we chose to live in denial for a while. Denial was a safe defense mechanism and spread like a contagious disease throughout my family and friends.

What we saw before us fueled our denial. Emma turned one on July 6, 2002. On her first birthday, we celebrated in a huge way, which was the polar opposite of Emma's tiny frame. We rented a gigantic water-slide and put it in the front yard. Emma slid down the slide with Eli and I. We had a house full of children and tons of presents.

She wasn't a typical one year old. She couldn't walk, sit up, or talk, but she was alert, friendly to everyone she met and she was meeting milestones very slowly. For months we continued with early intervention therapies and specialist appointments. Eli and I had faith that God had created her exactly in His image and we were so proud to be her parents.

By the time Emma was 18 months old she had a head full red curls, and she could gobble down peanut butter and jelly sandwiches and ice-cream. Cappuccino-flavored ice-cream was her favorite. She was capable of spotting food on the edge of the counter and, while sitting in her high chair, would maneuver her little body to snatch the food off the counter and shove it into her little mouth.

We rejoiced in her antics and every bit of spunk or advance Emma showed helped us to put aside any thoughts of a debilitating syndrome. Sure, she was tiny and delayed, but she couldn't have a debilitating, terminal syndrome like Cockayne, we rationalized.

Cockayne Syndrome is a genetic disease, and a form of advanced aging. Over time, it wreaks havoc on the children's bodies, but doesn't touch their personality, or their spunk.

My Journey with Emma

Despite my cocoon of denial, I always knew the truth. It lingered in that odd sense of knowing that lies within the depths of a mother. In my heart, I knew Emma had Cockayne Syndrome and would face an ugly, early, and terminal end.

I lived day to day, unable to imagine how devastating "the syndrome" would become. I believed the faces of the gaunt, elderly-looking children on the Cockayne Syndrome website would never be the face of my child.

Anne, the woman whose daughter Hannah had died at age four from Cockayne Syndrome, became my friend. She kept gently reminding me, "It is a degenerative syndrome." Still, my husband, in-laws, parents, and even myself to an extent, chose to keep pushing Anne away. She spoke too much truth for a family living steadfast in denial. Emma was just one and a half years old; she looked healthy and vivacious.

When Emma was nearing her second birthday, Eli and I decided to limit Emma's physical, speech, and occupational therapies. She experienced so much discomfort from these sessions we began to seek out alternative therapies. Instead of adhering to a strict regime of traditional therapies nine times a week, we chose a combination of traditional and alternative therapies and non-invasive ways of dealing with her physical and mental limitations.

Slowly, Emma began to meet milestones. She was always determined and paved her own way. She learned how to move herself around in a walker and had her own way of "sitting up." She never learned to talk, but we learned how to tell what she wanted. We taught her sign language and she was able to communicate in small ways through signing. Much to our delight, she could also be dramatic. She would throw her arms up into the air when she was done eating, and slam her hands on the highchair tray when she wanted more food.

Chapter 5 Intervention & Denial

Emma was opinionated. She continued physical therapy for the benefits it provided her muscles, but she would cry when she saw her physical therapist, Andrea, walk through the front door. Physical therapy was painful for Emma, but Andrea knew her well, and helped keep her tiny joints and muscles limber even though Emma screamed and tried to bite her. Every time Andrea would begin getting her things ready to leave, Emma would impatiently begin waving bye-bye, ready for the therapist to leave the house.

We taught Emma the song "The Itsy Bitsy Spider." The day she learned to clap, at almost two years old, I cried tears of joy and pride and called everyone to tell them the good news. Emma showed us how simple milestones can become hallmark events not only in her life, but in all of our lives.

Emma always had a sense of humor. She learned to roll on her side throughout the house to go wherever she wanted to go. She would roll under the couch to hide, and giggle when we couldn't find her. She fed herself cookies and cheerios and would beg for cappuccino-flavored ice cream every time she saw her daddy open the freezer door. She threw temper tantrums when other kids played with her toys, and when she didn't have her mommy's full attention. Finally, at two years old, she began to sleep through the night.

I'm Not Special

chapter six

*From My Journal
I trust in the Lord. All the days have already been planned.
It is my job to trust, have faith and pray. To love.
Not to change reality.*

The foundation of my life shook with the realization that my child had special needs. My own childhood was quite sheltered. My parents were overprotective and careful about what I was exposed to in the world. They did their best to protect me from tragedy, pain and grief.

I did experience the pain of my parent's divorce, but I believed my life as a mother would be similar to the perfect fairy tale existence I had conjured up in my mind about my future. I deserved clean, well- behaved children, and a beautiful home filled with perpetual sunlight. Reality hit hard as I found myself with a two-year-old son who thought he was Batman and could dive off the stairwell, and a tiny little daughter who didn't grow and seemed to fit the diagnosis for a terminal illness.

My reality did not fit in with the fantasy I had created in my mind since I was fourteen-years-old. I did not want the world to see that my house was always a mess, that I burned many meals because I was so distracted, or that I fed my children strawberry shortcake for dinner sometimes.

On the roughest days, I forgot to feed the cat and the dog. The cat would hurl herself at the backdoor meowing for food. My home was filled with Excel spreadsheets as I did my best to keep up with medications, therapies and doctor appointments for Emma.

I wished I were keeping up with the other moms I saw around me instead of the craziness. Those moms were toting their children to the park, grocery store, and story time. My days were mostly filled with therapies, doctors, and trying to keep my sanity intact. People would say things to me like, "Special kids are given to special people." Although it's a very kind sentiment, at the time it was frustrating to hear those words and I wanted to yell, "I don't want to be special!"

Those well-meaning comments created an expectation that I was some kind of wonder-mom. Along with my "specialness," there was pressure to do everything right. I had tremendous guilt whenever I felt overwhelmed, frustrated, or tired. The struggle to live up to the "special mommy" status bestowed on me became overwhelming.

I began to feel very different from other mothers and began to isolate, drawing inside of myself. As the others chatted and complained about their toddlers getting into typical messes, my heart yearned for Emma to be able do any of the things those other moms complained about.

I felt no one could comprehend my reality. My friend Amy had moved to another state and we were no longer in touch. I was desperate for friends and for understanding, but often felt judged. I even had to sever one friendship because the woman was so critical of the decisions I made concerning my family and children. I couldn't leave the house to go to Pilates with her in the evenings, and she became angry that I was not able to find time for my friendship with her. Dealing with her drama was not worth it.

I learned to survive without friends, and instead surrounded myself with my family. My kids and husband were my entire world. Peyton, Emma and I went everywhere together. Peyton and Emma were best

CHAPTER 6 — I'm Not Special

friends. Peyton doted on his little sister, and she adored him. To him, Emma never had special needs, mental retardation, microcephaly, or failure to thrive. She was never the product of a genetic mutation. In Peyton's world, Emma was just his little sister.

And that is how it was for all of us, our entire family. We weren't special. We were just us. We lived and loved, no matter what was going on. In the center of it all, God increased in magnitude in my mind. He became my eternal hope, and the source of my strength.

When Emma was a year and a half old, we found out our daughter Paige was on her way. We didn't know if she would be born with Cockayne Syndrome or not. We still didn't have a firm diagnosis for Emma, and we certainly didn't have a terminal diagnosis for her either.

While pregnant with Paige I began to meet with a group of women from a church support group. Every week those women listened to my cries of fear, anxiety, and hope for the child growing within me. In that group of loving women, I found safety expressing my deepest fears. I voiced my fear of the reality that Emma would not live much longer, and my worries that the child I was carrying would be born having the same condition as Emma. Paige will probably never fully understand the circumstances surrounding her birth or how deeply we prayed over her.

The women in my support group enveloped me in a protective web of faith, love and hope. They wrapped me in circles of prayer, and prayed over my unborn child, Paige. They prayed to God for her to be born healthy. They prayed for our family to accept with comfort everything that the future would bring. They prayed for peace in all that was to come.

My hope did not come from believing that Emma would improve, but instead it came as my understanding of God's grace increased. The wells of darkness I had fallen into during Emma's first year of life became filled with light. The sadness and bitterness I once felt lifted from my soul.

Every morning, I wrapped Emma up with song, prayer, and adoration to God. As my pregnancy continued and the calendar grew closer to my due date, the Lord quieted my fears. I had an overwhelming realization that it would be okay regardless of if Paige was born healthy, or if she had the same condition as Emma.

Emma turned two on a sweltering-hot July day. We celebrated by having a party with a Pooh Bear cake and ice-cream. That morning, I gave Emma a bath and dressed her in her cutest outfit: tiny little Capri pants, sized for a six-month-old.

As I sat her in her highchair to snap photos of her, I stopped and absorbed the happy grin on her face. I took note of her porcelain skin and bright blue eyes, all framed by strawberry blonde hair that hung in long curls. She looked so healthy and happy. I turned to get Eli's attention, and we both stood in front of our daughter gazing at her.

"Isn't she beautiful, Eli?" I asked.

"She is. She is our 'Little Bit' of love," he replied with pride. "Happy Birthday, Little Bit!"

Emma sat in her high chair and fed herself gobs of cake and ice-cream all by herself. She wore a pointy birthday hat featuring a giant Pooh Bear, and grinned happily at us covered in yellow icing.

She tore open her birthday presents and squealed when she saw the gifts. It was an almost unbelievable scene. Just a year before, we never thought she would be able to sit in a highchair, eat independently, or be aware of her surroundings.

But on that second birthday she was at her peak, and we were encouraged. She was a tiny, tiny little girl, but she seemed to be doing so well. The happy memory of her sitting in that highchair grinning as Eli and I gazed at her will stay with me forever. At the same time,

CHAPTER 6 I'm ~~Not~~ Special

we had another child about to be born in four months, and it was very frightening knowing she might have the same syndrome Emma did.

The Lord continued to care for our family and the children He blessed our home with. During my pregnancy with Paige I felt God drawing me closer to Him. I began to trust the Lord more than ever before. In hindsight, I am able to see His work over and over again in our lives. When I prayed for a strong support system, God encircled me with the body of Christ and people who truly cared for us.

I learned that with every storm of our life, there are blessings too. During this time, the Lord led me to Ezekiel 34:26, "I will send down showers in season; there will be showers of blessing." I learned that maybe I was wrong, maybe this whole time I was special. I certainly have been a blessed, special daughter of the King.

Emma at her 2nd Birthday Party

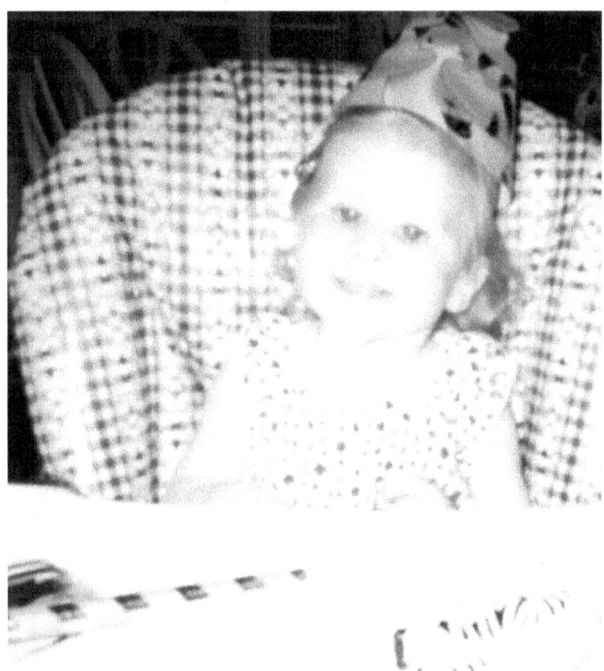

Out of the Darkness

chapter seven

"Only when we are no longer afraid do we begin to live."
—Dorothy Thompson

A few months after her second birthday, Emma quit eating. She started losing her eyesight, and her face began to look gaunt. Her hair started thinning. The strawberry blonde curls, which had once hung down her back, became a memory.

After living in a safe bubble of denial for a year, Eli and I still clung to the hope that we would find Emma's true diagnosis. And we prayed it would *not* be the terminal Cockayne Syndrome that Anne and the Houston doctor had suggested to us. Emma couldn't have Cockayne Syndrome. We refused to wake from our sweet slumber of denial.

Not only did I live with my own denial, I had to live with family members' denial. One of the most difficult tasks I had to do was to tell Eli's mother about Emma's likely diagnosis.

"Emma might have a degenerative brain disease," I exhaled in desperation as I explained the details of Emma's previous brain scans to my mother-in-law.

She looked at me, put her hands on her hips and said, "Well, we will just see about that."

After that, I didn't mention it again. But even then, in my heart, I knew Emma had the syndrome. I just couldn't bear to utter the words. My family's denial was quite intense. Simply mentioning Cockayne

Syndrome would result in sighs and rolling eyes. Denial was the way we all survived reality.

"That Anne woman makes you paranoid," family members would say. But Anne was my friend whose daughter had passed away from Cockayne's. I didn't like what she had to say, but I needed her in my life.

None of us wanted to believe we would ever have to live without looking into the eyes of a child we loved. We saw hope in Emma's eyes. That was one truth we each fought to hold on to.

But even with all of our hope, we still couldn't deny Emma's symptoms. There was definitely a problem. Still searching for answers, Eli and I reluctantly made the decision to put Emma through *one more test*.

We discovered a test that would hopefully bring us the diagnosis we wanted to hear—amino acid deficiency. Emma fit many of the criteria for the diagnosis. We found a research company that did testing for amino acid deficiencies. We completed the paperwork, scheduled an appointment and prayed for a miracle.

Very early one fall morning, just as dawn began to light the sky, I drove Emma to the hospital for them to draw spinal fluid. Even though she was medicated, it wasn't enough to keep her from being afraid. It was excruciating to hear her muffled screams as the medical staff drew the precious fluid from her tiny spine. She was just a little girl, but they had to hold her down to perform the procedure.

I was still pregnant with Paige. My hormones were raging. My raw emotions brimmed over and I sobbed uncontrollably, wishing I could take Emma's pain away. There was nothing I could do but listen to her cry. The nurses steered me out of the room when they saw my giant belly and sobbing face.

During Emma's spinal tap, I watched from a distance as I leaned on a hospital bed that was randomly in the hallway outside of her room.

Chapter 7 *Out of the Darkness*

It seemed to have been a mistake to put her through the procedure. I never wanted to see my baby in pain, especially when it was my choice to do the test.

A month passed and, before we learned what mysteries Emma's spinal fluid revealed, our third child Paige was born November 21, 2003. She weighed in at nearly ten pounds with a head full of brown hair, and little fat rolls on her body. She was completely healthy, and we rejoiced! Oh, how we rejoiced!

Eli and I prayed that the good fortune of our third child being born healthy would spread over to Emma's awaited test results, and that she would be with us forever.

My most profound point of change—coming out of the darkness of denial—came on the day I answered a phone call from the neurologist. She had the test results. In dark contrast to the vibrant fall colors outside our home, my internal world completely drained of color as I listened to Dr. Teasley's words.

I remember the conversation I had with Eli after I hung up the phone.

"Dr. Teasley just called with the results. Emma's spinal fluid has high levels of protein. She has a degenerative brain disease, most likely Cockayne Syndrome, not the amino acid deficiency like we'd hoped."

Eli's face became pale. His strong physical veneer crushed. His whole body shook as he gazed at Emma from across the room. She was happily giggling at her older brother, Peyton.

Both of us were trapped in a quiet, immobile moment as we internally careened out of control. I could feel his paralyzing fear as he asked me the question that the rest of our life with Emma centered around.

"Is she going to die?" Eli had finally conceded his little girl was very sick.

"Yes, but not today, not tomorrow, and not next week," I said.

"What are we going to do?" he asked. I wanted to console him, to cushion him from the crashing fall I knew he was taking.

"We are going to live life, have fun, laugh, and make each day we have left with her a memory," I said.

And we did.

We absorbed our children's squealing laughter. We took part in their games with pure childlike joy. Eli and I were united in our acceptance of Emma's disease. We were no longer blinded by denial.

If I could recapture a time to return to, it would be that autumn. The timing of her diagnosis was perfect because we were able to enjoy a beautiful season with Emma before she started growing weaker. Peyton, Emma and Paige—all three of our children were with us. It was just before the hands of time began to spin faster, and faster.

After our time of joy and laughter, we entered a season where calendars don't exist and where time whirls like a missile spinning toward its target—our daughter's earthly existence. Emma was lingering on an invisible stairwell, about to begin her slow decent. This season was the quiet eerie calm that comes before a torrential storm.

I began to see the triviality in most of life's problems. I also began to fully understand the importance of laughter. I learned that life is not measured by time, but by the joy we absorb from the ones we love, and the joy they receive from the love we give back.

Love doesn't need a voice. I found love in the unspoken gaze of my child who was never able to speak a word. It is that kind of love that conquers all fear of the future.

A Wish Come True

chapter eight

"Every life is touched by miracles. Sometimes people just don't recognize them, but that doesn't mean that what they are experiencing is not a miracle."
—Henri Landwirth, Founder, Give Kids the World

Emma was two-years-old when I started seeing commercials popping up on television about a place called *Give Kids the World*. It was a whimsical resort created to give children with a terminal illness a fun vacation. I put *Give Kids the World* into my mental filing cabinet many months before Emma's official diagnosis. It seemed like a place my family was destined to visit someday.

Emma's clinical diagnosis of Cockayne Syndrome came after the spinal testing for amino acid problems. Doctors compared what they saw in her blood results with what they knew about Cockayne Syndrome. Eventually, we began to see Cockayne's in her face. The once elusive syndrome made its name very evident in our lives, and we had no choice but to accept it.

After Emma's diagnosis, I called *Magic Moments*—a wish-granting organization, which ran out of Children's Hospital in Birmingham. I uncontrollably sobbed as I spoke to Evelyn, the wish coordinator, about a wish for Emma. Evelyn was patient, compassionate, and assured me that *Magic Moments* would do everything possible to make Emma's wish come true. Hearing her say that was another truth pervading my life. My child had a terminal illness, and was eligible for a "wish."

We had to find out what Emma's wish was, even though she could not speak. As always, in her own way, Emma let us know exactly what she wanted.

Emma loved Mickey Mouse. When I was a child, my aunt Gale gave me a giant stuffed Mickey Mouse. It was a prize from her trip to Disney World. I passed the giant stuffed Mickey Mouse down to my children. Emma would squeal when she saw Mickey. She grabbed his nose, delight shining on her face as she laughed hysterically.

Emma also loved it when Peyton would dress up in superhero costumes—Superman, Batman, or any other hero. He would "fly" through the house in a whirlwind of boy-energy. As he ran, he came to a halt near Emma. Peyton would put his hands on his hips, and spread out his legs in a wide stance in front of her. Then he would absorb the laugh that was sure to ensue from her tiny frame.

We combined Emma's love of Mickey and her joy at seeing her brother dressed in costumes and came up with her wish. Although she could not speak the words, we knew she would love to meet Mickey and see all the characters at Disney World.

Magic Moments required children to be four-years-old to have a wish granted, but magically, they granted Emma's wish when she was three. The staff at the organization knew Emma's time was short, and she may not live to be four-years-old. Emma was going to meet Mickey Mouse and get to stay at *Give Kids the World* for a week!

It took a few months after we found out Emma's wish would be granted for us to be ready to go. We had to wait for flu season to pass, and get through Christmas. Emma went on hospice care, and we knew it was time to take her to *Give Kids the World*.

We took oxygen tanks, the hospice telephone numbers, and pain medications with us. Somehow, the magic of Emma's wish spilled over and her health improved while we were in Florida. She was alert and

CHAPTER 8 *A Wish Come True*

filled with excitement. She ventured out each day to experience a new adventure.

We watched Emma laugh at Buzz Lightyear, Stitch, Donald Duck, Goofy, and many other Disney characters. When the staff at Disney World saw Emma's name badge and the words *Give Kids the World*, they treated her like royalty. Staff members moved us to the front of every line. Compassionate people dressed in costume would stop for several minutes to spend time with Emma while other people patiently waited in line to get the characters' autographs. It seemed like Emma caused time to stand still for these wonderful people who showed her love.

Every person at Disney appeared to know how special a girl Emma was. Winnie the Pooh even scooped her into his arms when he met her. Emma was peaceful, and our entire family felt like a fairy had sprinkled pixie dust all over us.

Then Emma met Mickey Mouse. We watched our tiny Emma look up in wonder at him. She reached out to gently touch Mickey's nose as if to make sure he was real and she wasn't in a dream. The smile, which spread across her face as her wish was fulfilled, told us we made the right choice. Going to Disney World and *Give Kids the World* was exactly what Emma wanted.

Emma with her Daddy, Eli

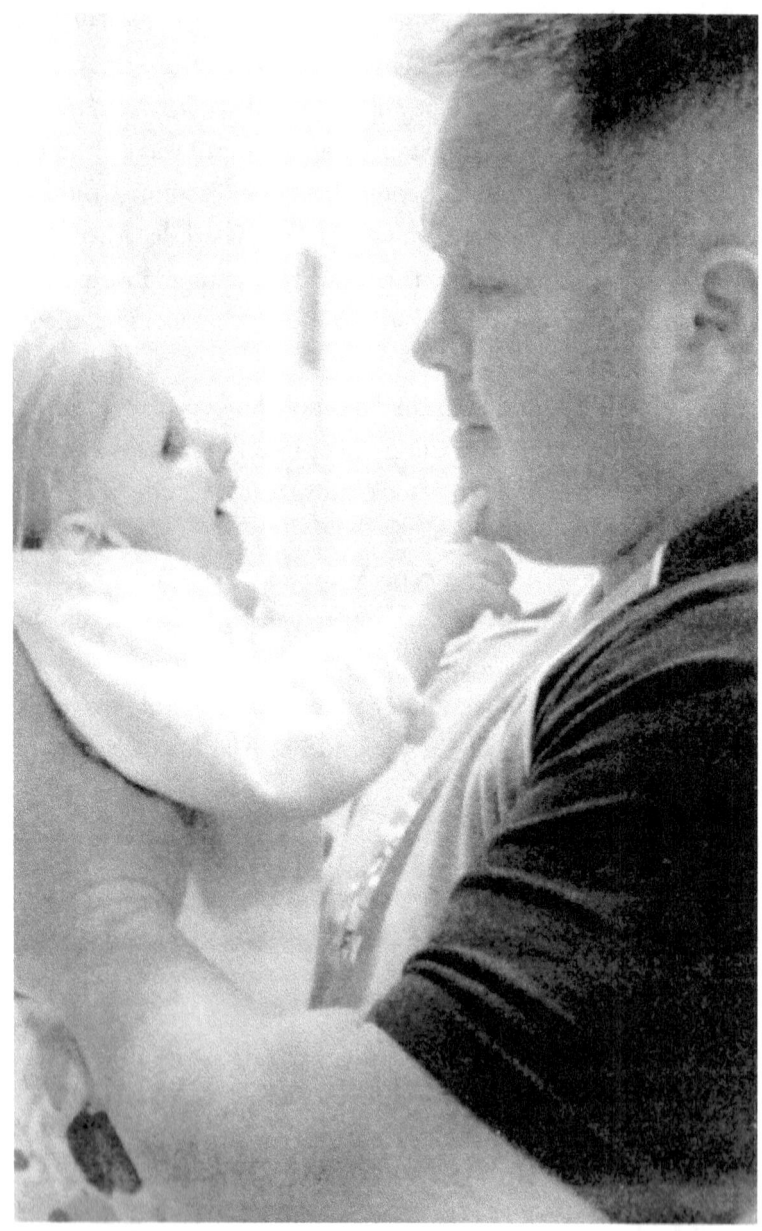

Decline

chapter nine

From My Journal
"Through suffering, we come to know joy. My hope is in the Lord that whatever the future may hold, all answers are in Him. To know Him and to learn His ways will bring peace."

The winter after her second birthday, Emma started declining at a more rapid pace. In just six months, she started looking gaunt and began losing skills she once had. We watched our once bubbly and active child become exhausted and uninterested in toys. The saddest part for me was when she stopped rolling through the house. That was always her favorite mode of "transportation." As she grew weaker, it seemed as if I were caring for a little, elderly lady. Dark circles surrounded her once bright eyes, and she began to refuse food and drink.

Every few months, I would move another piece of equipment—her walker, her stander, her special chair—to the corner of the room. It would sit and begin gathering dust. Eventually, I moved the equipment into the garage, never to return to our home. Emma was too weak to use any of it anymore. I kept holding onto hope that she would become stronger and be able to stand up again, that one day she would reach for her baby sister.

But she didn't.

Our safe cocoon of denial was gone. Eli and I began to have to make painful decisions concerning Emma's care. As the syndrome advanced, Emma became weaker. We consulted with therapists, doctors, and even alternative medicine. We did everything we could think of to help extend her life. It was to no avail. She continued to decline.

My dad and stepmom came to visit us after Paige was born, which was around the time of Emma's diagnosis. When they saw Emma's frail frame, the looks on their faces showed sheer despair. The whole week during their visit, they were trying to get Emma to eat.

What we didn't understand was that Emma wasn't capable of eating like a typical child. No matter what we fed her, she wasn't able to maintain calories. On one visit to the pediatrician's office, I begged the doctor to listen to me. I told her we were doing everything we could to get calories into Emma's body, but she would clamp her mouth shut and refuse food. If she did eat, she would end up throwing up.

Meals became a battlefield. Emma seemed afraid to eat, perhaps because she connected eating with the inevitable act of throwing up. We gave her ice-cream along with food the doctors recommended, which included thickening her food and giving her Carnation instant breakfast shakes.

We were desperate to help her, but the pediatrician's recommendations were not viable solutions. Emma was always so tiny and never weighed over 14 pounds. Now, even with her small size, she began to look emaciated. The skin around her tummy began wrinkling and sagging.

At another appointment, I overheard Emma's pediatrician in the hallway asking the nurse to get the gastroenterologist to find time to see Emma before our scheduled appointment.

"This is a child on the edge," I heard the doctor say. I was afraid to ask or even contemplate what "edge" he was referring to.

We eventually consulted with the gastroenterologist about placing a feeding tube into Emma's stomach, and it happened in February 2004. Even with the feeding tube, Emma never weighed more than

Chapter 9 Decline

14-15 pounds, but once she had it we could give her food continuously at intervals throughout the day and night. It helped her tiny tummy to digest smaller amounts of food, retain nutrients, and reduce the amount of throwing up.

Over the next year, Emma regained some energy, but was continued on a downward decent as she lost skills. The pattern continued until we had to make the decision to place her on hospice in December 2004.

Emma taught us unconditional love. Each time she declined—requiring new medication, oxygen, and eventually hospice—we would unconditionally accept it, just as we accepted and embraced Emma. It was never a sacrifice to care for her. I would have happily taken care of her for the rest of my life.

She was my "Little Bit," like a koala bear always in my arms. The truth is, the whole time I was holding Emma, God was working on my faith through my baby. He was the one carrying me.

Introspective

It was a Wednesday. Emma had been under hospice care for nearly six months. I was in a hurry and had Peyton in the car. We were headed to his preschool. He was his usual introspective, yet active self. On the way to school, Peyton asked me a question. He had been quiet that morning, which was unusual for him.

"Mommy, when is Emma going to die?" He asked.

I held my breath as my mind raced to find an age-appropriate answer for my barely five-year-old son.

I glanced at the mountains lining the landscape and noticed the beautiful May morning sunlight as it beat down on the windshield of our suburban. I found myself contemplating truth and wondering how to answer his profound question.

How many preschoolers have to worry about their little sister dying? I pondered. *Why does my son have to live through this? God, please give me words!*

Finally, I replied, "I don't know, Honey. Only God knows that answer."

"Mommy, is it soon that Emma will be able to run?" He asked me pointedly.

I absorbed the impact of what my little boy said. He said "run." Run. At that moment, Peyton knew more than I did. Emma had never been able to take a single step, or walk at all, yet, he was aware that she would soon be able to run.

My brain, body, and soul went weak, but God took over my spirit. After a long exhale and pause, I said, "Yes, I think so, Buddy. Emma is very, very weak now."

I hated to say that. I hated to admit defeat, loss of control, and inevitable death. I hated to admit the truth.

Childlike, full of innocence and love, Peyton said to me, "I'm glad God made Emma my little sister. I think Emma will be happy to run."

I found truth in Peyton's innocence. In that quiet moment, I felt relief, heartache, and peace all at the same time. Peyton knew Emma was going to die. He knew that her death was coming soon, and he was processing it much quicker than I was. God was already giving him a sense of peace through the middle of everything. It would take me years to absorb that peace.

Walking Through the Shadow

chapter ten

"Emma was loved by so many people. I will never forget how beautiful she was and will think about her every day. I put one of my Livestrong bracelets into her casket because that is how Emma lived, strong. She was a tough little fighter who touched people."
—Uncle Wes

My Journal – April 4, 2005

Emma girl,

You are so sick with pneumonia right now. We are struggling to capture your smiles, your sounds and your scent.

You will get better, I believe that. But I am so scared.

There are many choices we have had to make about your care. The most important thing is to keep you comfortable, but sometimes you cry all night and seem to be in tremendous pain. I'm in pain for you, and unable to take your pain away.

My friend Jackie came from Virginia to help take care of you. It was such a blessing to have her here for a few days.

What a paradox of life. We have oxygen tanks, wires running throughout the house, and nursing sheets tracking multiple medications. In an attempt to keep you hydrated, we are running your g-tube with small amounts of fluid 24-hours a day.

In stark contrast, we have a 17-month-old toddler perfecting her walking as she tip-toes through the oxygen tank wiring. She has learned what buttons to push on your g-tube machine when it begins

My Journey with Emma

beeping. Like a tiny, compassionate nurse Paige peers at you, pats you, and alerts us when something needs to be fixed with the feeding machine.

We have a 5-year-old son who is running around like Batman through the house, seemingly oblivious to all that is going on. I asked Peyton what he thought about the wires, the medicines, your bed in the living room, and the hospice nurses coming in daily. He replied "It's just Emma." Peyton has always accepted you just as you are. For your entire life, he has continued to have an intuitive connection to you, an awareness which defies any earthly explanation.

My Journal – Late April, 2005

Emma Catherine,

You are a strong little girl. You just recovered from a scary pneumonia. It happened so quickly. Even though you are on hospice, we had to decide whether we would hospitalize you, put IV's in you, and possibly put you on a breathing machine. We ultimately decided to keep you home, under hospice care.

We held you, gave you your breathing treatments, and trusted in the Lord. I believe we made the right decision. Next time, it could be worse. We don't want you to go through a hospitalization. We just want you to be home where you are the most comfortable.

You have recovered and have begun smiling at us. You are laughing again and we delight in your happy squeals. We love to hold you and have your little arms wrap around our necks. You have returned to us!

So many have prayed for you. You touch all of their lives. You say no words, but speak to every heart that listens to you. They see God in your eyes, and in your spirit.

Chapter 10 — Walking Through the Shadow

Sometimes I think you are the bravest of us all. You are trying to tell us it is OK. As I learn more about my own faith I am less afraid of what the future holds. For now, I love to hold you, and have you look at me and touch my face. You fall asleep curled so close to me and I am absorbing watching you breathe so softly.

I love you Little Bit,
Mommy

May 22, 2005

Three hours before Emma died, I knelt at her bedside and in a barely audible voice whispered to her.

"Emma, I don't want to say this to you because I want you to stay with me, but I love you, and I know you are very tired and sick. If you are ready to leave, then I want you to know it is OK.

I will be fine. Daddy will take care of Mommy, Mommy will take care of Daddy, and we will see you again."

The look on her face showed understanding and she exhaled a sigh of relief. Her eyes said a silent, "Thank you."

She closed her cloudy blue eyes and slept for the next two hours. She hadn't been able to sleep for the past 48-hours, but finally my words comforted her enough to sleep. She had relapsed into another more aggressive pneumonia a mere week earlier. This time, we knew she would not recover.

I was too antsy to rest. Instead, I sat watching her breathing, afraid to leave her. My friend Patti stayed at the house the night before and left around 5 a.m. It was now 6 a.m. I sat on the couch near Emma, trapped in a state of immobile silence.

Eli, Peyton, and Paige were upstairs sleeping. Peyton woke up around 7 a.m. and asked to hold his sister. I took pictures of them together. Peyton looked scared. Instinctively, he knew Emma was going to run and dance soon. He still wanted to hold her, to make her feel better.

Her breaths were shallow. The oxygen stayed attached to her, and I was giving her breathing treatments every two hours. Hospice nurses came into our home numerous times during the previous 24-hours. We knew her body was in the final stage of life on earth.

I called Eli's parent's who lived just down the street, as well as my dad who was 500 miles away in Texas.

"I think you need to get here as soon as you can," I told both sets of grandparents. I couldn't call my mom. I didn't know how to tell her the truth. There had been so much pain in her life. How could I tell her Emma was about to leave us? She was heartbroken for Emma, and for me.

Eli's parents came to our house immediately. They wanted to hold her. Emma seemed peaceful and comfortable, so I rushed to get dressed and hurried back downstairs.

As I rounded the corner into the living room my mother-in-law, Cecile, said, "She just sat up in Russell's lap, smiled, and laughed at Peyton and Paige dancing."

HOPE! I thought. She would beat this pneumonia. A child about to die doesn't sit up and laugh.

Emma began to moan and reached for me. Russell looked horrified and said, "She wants you."

She passed away in my arms few moments later. Her heart gave way to the syndrome which caused advanced aging, and pneumonia. Finally, she was able to dance.

I stared at her. Peace enveloped her face. I looked into her eyes. They were as clear as the sky on a spring morning. She was entering her new home, taking her first steps, seeing life in full color now, I knew.

Chapter 10: Walking Through the Shadow

My friend Sandra arrived on my doorstep that morning, after she heard God telling her to go to our home instead of church. Our dear Kari went to get my mother, and bring her to our home so we could tell her in person Emma was dying.

Wind chimes sang as they clanged together on the front porch. I sat in shock, holding Emma, unable to move. Jan, our hospice nurse arrived immediately. Still seated in the chair holding Emma, I looked up at Jan and whispered, "I was going to give her a bath today."

She said, "Well let's do that then. I will help you."

Jan helped me to bathe Emma one last time. Her body was frail. Jan was filled with compassion and allowed me to bathe my daughter.

I bathed her in the bathtub I'd always bathed her in, and then I laid her down on Eli's and my bed to dress her in her little pair of pink pajamas.

When I laid her down, she was so peaceful. I didn't need to worry about a feeding tube as I dressed her. My entire focus was on bathing and dressing my baby for the last time. I was trying to absorb all the emotion that held.

It was the last time I would ever hold my child here on earth. I dressed her, combed her hair, and fussed over her. I did it all in a state of shock, I suppose.

My dear friends Patti and Jennifer helped me cut locks of Emma's hair to keep, and they helped me to make her tiny handprint.

After she was bathed and dressed in her pajamas, Eli stood in Emma's room, holding her. He was sobbing, and refused to walk down the stairs with her.

"I can't leave the house with her. I just can't let her go," he said.

"She is already gone," I said. "We have to do this now. Taking her downstairs is the next part of the journey." He looked at me with tears falling down his strong face, and agreed. I took Emma from his arms, and we walked together down the stairs and out of our home. She was wrapped in her pink blanket, and her hair still held the lingering scent of baby shampoo.

The people from the funeral home waited outside. I handed Emma over to a man dressed in a suit. He held her gently in his arms and climbed into the passenger side of the SUV hearse. He held her all the way to the funeral home.

A peaceful breeze swept over Eli and me as we stood watching the hearse move slowly down the street taking our daughter away from our home forever.

> *"So we are always of good courage. We know that while we are at home in the body we are away from the Lord, for we walk by faith, not by sight. Yes, we are of good courage, and we would rather be away from the body and at home with the Lord."* 2 Corinthians 5:6-8

The morning after Emma left her earthly home, I woke early, showered, and prepared for the most horrifying week of my life. In a couple of hours, we would have to go to the funeral home and cemetery to make arrangements for Emma's burial. As I walked down the stairs into our living room, there was still a hint of normalcy.

Emma's tiny, temporary bed we kept downstairs was still in the corner. There sat the oxygen tanks, the tubing coiled neatly around the pump gages. Her medications were still in the refrigerator. She was the only thing missing.

Exhaling, I sank into the chair I had held her in less than 24-hours earlier as she took her last breath. Sobbing, I bowed my head and began to pray.

"Thank you, Lord, for this journey, for my beautiful, exquisite Emma. We are blessed and grateful to You for trusting us with her

CHAPTER 10 — Walking Through the Shadow

tender care. We know she is safe in Your loving arms, free from the pain she was in. Lord, please help me to know what to do now. The last three and a half years my life centered on her care. What do I do now, on this morning, the first morning of the rest of my life without my Little Bit? What do I do?"

As I continued to bow, pray, and sob, I heard a gentle voice say, "Just play. Just play with Peyton and Paige. Enjoy them, and pour all that energy you gave to Emma into them now."

Smiling through the tears as I lifted my head, I said, "Thank You." I rose from the chair and went to wake my children, wrapping them in my arms and repeating over and over, "I love you."

We were a family of five with three children, one with terminal needs. Suddenly, we were a family of four, seemingly, to the outside world, a typical family. But we were not. We had been through pain many families do not have to face. We were like a whole different family now.

We began the rest of our life with Peyton and Paige that day.

Release

Family and friends gathered near a small maple tree in the historic cemetery. Emma's tiny white casket was the focal point, garnished with colorful flowers and silk butterflies.

A few members of our church's praise team began to sing "Blessed Be the Name of the Lord." As their voices filled the small tent and filtered out to the crowd, I heard everyone around me slowly start singing in unison. The words of the song rose up to Heaven in a beautiful wave of worship.

You give and take away. You give and take away. My heart will choose to say, Lord, blessed be Your Name . . .

My Journey with *Emma*

As the service ended, Eli, Peyton and I gathered together and slowly lifted the lid off a small white box filled with monarch butterflies. One by one, each butterfly stretched it's wings and fluttered up into the air.

One landed on my dad's hand and rested for a while, before beginning its journey. Emma's funeral was a celebration of life, as beautiful as the time she spent on earth.

Truth from my Tiny

chapter eleven

"She had a way of making you fall in love with her from the very first moment. The beauty of her smile will forever shine in my heart. She will have the angels wrapped around her little finger. Thank you for sharing Emma with us. We are more loving and accepting because we had both you and Emma to teach us. Your strength through this has amazed me. I know it comes from the Lord. Celebrate her life. When pain comes, rejoice in her smile and the moments she made your heart light up. The brightest star in the night—that's our Emma."
—Ms. Laura, Emma's preschool teacher

One month after Emma passed away, feelings of regret and many questions consumed my brain. Did I do enough? Did I make the right decisions? Where did I go wrong in her care? Why couldn't I do enough for her to keep her here, at least for another year?

Eli would remind me that we made decisions together. God created Emma and decided when it was time for her to go. Eli helped me to remember that we did make the right decisions. We did make Emma happy, and we kept her healthy for as long as we were able to.

Despite the truth Eli reminded me of, I still had an overwhelming feeling that I was entirely responsible for Emma's life and death. I was the one who carried her in my body, delivered her, got up all night with her, and experimented with diets, supplements, and therapies. Throughout Emma's life, I did the research to find what foods, supplements, and therapies would make her healthier. I felt responsible. I felt guilty. My head felt swollen with the thought that I hadn't done enough to keep Emma here.

Despite my battle with guilt and regret, I know the truth is that I did do enough to keep Emma happy, smiling, and joyous. I held her. I spoiled her. I doted on her. I took care of Emma with joy. I loved her.

Even when exhaustion set in, I kept going, getting up at night with her just to hold her when she was uncomfortable, throwing up, and having nerve pain. Sometimes she would cry for days on end. I didn't become angry or frustrated with her. I just took care of her. She would lie in my arms, moan and fidget for hours. Eventually, she would fall asleep as I held her, and I would fall asleep too. I cherish those times. Through it all, I knew she wouldn't be here for long, and knew it would be painful to lose her. I never knew how much it would ache to miss holding her, though. I miss her so much it physically hurts.

Even though I grieve for her, and my heart aches, I would care for her over again. Even though I knew her precious life would end much too soon, Emma was a miracle. She was an amazing child who aged faster than her parents did.

After Emma died, people would ask, "How are you doing?"

That first week after she died, my answer was, "I'm walking." It was the best answer I could muster. I simply walked like a robot through those early days. Taking care of my children, my husband, and myself was all I could do. Thankfully, my role as wife and mommy has always been firmly imprinted in my being, and my family was enough motivation to make it easy to wake up, get out of bed, and start the day.

Then reality would set in. Emma wasn't here. I didn't need to fill her feeding bags, monitor the medications, or make calls to hospice. We no longer had the task of reordering supplies or filling out forms for medical reimbursements. Emma's life with us in this realm was over. We didn't need to be concerned about her reflux, joint stiffness, stretching, or finding toys that would excite her, or make her smile.

CHAPTER 11 — Truth from my Tiny

Space and time converged and I wandered around in a fog-like existence. It was hard to see the outline of anything outside of my immediate view. Staring into space took precedent over dirty diapers, bills, and dishes. Life was simply walking, or stumbling, from one event to another. Looking back, I can see that shock is necessary to survival during the initial stages of grief.

The grief journey is a like phantom, always there, sometimes revealing itself. I traveled through those early days, unsure of when a twisting turn would catch me off guard. Grief was mysterious. I did not know when the bottom would fall out of my nearly full bucket. Unexpectedly, the momentum of emotion would build up so much that my stomach would be in my throat, and I was incapable of conversation. I would seem to be making progress, doing well, then the panic attacks would come. I would sob painfully, so very aware of the reality that Emma was not coming back.

I tried to keep my emotions from Peyton and Paige, but Peyton was so perceptive. He would crawl in bed beside me and whisper, "Mommy, I'm so sorry you are sad. I miss her too. Do you want to hug a doll to make you feel better?"

My little boy's genuine attempt to comfort me in a profound sadness did make me smile. Eli and I held onto our children and made sure to take care of their grief as well. Peyton was old enough to go to grief counseling through the children's program at our hospice.

We all had an acute awareness of the emptiness in our home. Emma's absence was heightened by the awareness of how much my children missed her, and how the pain of grief seeped into every facet of our lives.

Strangely, in the midst of grief, I never asked, "Why?"

Yes, I wondered if I did enough, or if I did something wrong, but I never wondered why it all had to happen. I haven't questioned God's reason for bringing Emma here. She taught me so much. I don't think it is possible for me to share the depth of value Emma brought into my life.

I began to focus on God's sovereignty. I stopped taking responsibility for Emma's life and focused on God's power. I could not have changed the number of days Emma was on earth. It was in God's hands. I came to realize that no one else, including me, could love my daughter with the great measure of love God has for her. And she is in Heaven with Him now.

The knowledge of God has given me quietness in my soul, and peace about Emma not being here. My connection with my Father in heaven comforts my grief. I know He created Emma perfectly because of His love for her. I can't even fathom the depths of His love for her, and all of us.

Grief speaks many languages. Grief is raw, flesh-filled, emotional, and physically tormenting. After Emma died, I wrestled with guilt, anger, sadness, depression, regret, shock, and wanting to change the past.

As the battle of the flesh raged, God continued to whisper to me. May 22, 2005, was not a mistake. It was not a consequence of inadequate care, or any decision I made. It was the day that God brought peace to a little girl, and a day that made the heavens sing with delight. The morning Emma left us was the day her life began.

The Butterfly

chapter twelve

"What the caterpillar calls the end of the world, the Master calls a butterfly." —Richard Bach

"By faith we understand that the universe was formed at God's command, so that what is seen was not made out of what was visible." Hebrews 11:3

Emma's butterfly-shaped headstone is the only one in the historic cemetery where her body rests. Inscribed on Emma's headstone is the quote, "The butterfly counts not months, but moments, and has time enough."

Emma's life was much like a butterfly—a symbol of rebirth, renewal, fragility, and beauty. Yes, butterflies are here for only a short while, but they have time enough to teach, love, learn, and absorb all they need to in life.

After Emma passed away, butterflies seemed to flourish in front of my eyes in a way I had never seen before. They dipped and danced all throughout our backyard, and we saw them fluttering in places we never noticed them. Butterflies emerged not only in Eli's and my life, but in my parents' lives as well.

Butterflies now adorn our home. We have them on wind chimes, figurines, photographs, and lamps. Butterflies touch all of our lives in some way. It seems the Lord always sends a special Emma-butterfly at the times we need them the most.

One day, I looked out of my kitchen window and absorbed the graceful dance of a butterfly. The butterfly should not have been there. The temperatures had been below freezing, too low for a butterfly to survive in our North Alabama winter climate. Amazingly, a monarch butterfly appeared on that cold November day, fluttering around for me to see just after I received a phone call letting me know another child with Cockayne Syndrome had died.

Butterflies, it seemed, were something we needed to pay attention to. I began to research how butterflies were spiritually meaningful. I discovered they have amazing sight! They can see things we humans cannot, like ultraviolet light, which helps guide them to find nectar.

My faith guides me toward God, like the way butterflies are guided to nectar. As a believer in Christ, I see with eyes of faith. The human eye can't see my faith in God, but my faith is very real to me. As we walk by faith, we move forward toward God in a way others cannot see or understand.

Hebrews 11 offers examples of people who relied on faith in God even when the end result was not visible, and even when others mocked them. God warned Noah about events humans could not see. In obedience, Noah constructed an ark to save his family and others. By his faithful obedience, he became an heir of righteousness.

By faith, Abraham, when called to go to a place he would later receive as his inheritance, obeyed and went, even though he did not know where he was going. He was looking forward to a city whose architect and builder is God.

By faith, Moses, when he had grown up, refused to be known as the son of Pharaoh's daughter. He chose to be mistreated along with the people of God rather than to enjoy the pleasures of sin for a short time. By faith, he left Egypt, not fearing the king's anger; he persevered because he followed an invisible God who manifested in many ways.

By faith, we understand that everything we see (and everything we cannot see) was created by the Word of God, so that what is seen is "not made out of things that are visible."

Chapter 12 — The Butterfly

By faith, I know that while I cannot see or touch my daughter, she is very much alive in the Kingdom of Heaven, dancing in the presence of God—fluttering like a beautiful butterfly. Emma dances in the light of the Lord, and she is surely more alive than I am right now.

I like to think Emma is growing up in heaven, but I don't know. Maybe she will still be three years old, waiting for us to arrive to watch her grow up.

Either way, I know we will be with her again. When we see Jesus, all the pain we felt on earth will evaporate. Like a mother seeing her child for the first time, joy will overcome pain.

Heaven feels like a much closer place when you have a child there, when you know Jesus is there waiting for you, holding her hand. The colors in my world are bright, but I know the most vivid colors will come in the future in my heavenly life. Heaven is a place where there is only joy and peace. In Heaven, Eli and I will be reunited with our daughter.

On our 13th wedding anniversary weekend, we went on a little getaway. It was relaxing and peaceful, but I could not find fulfillment or calm. At that time, I felt it was too soon to let go of my thoughts of Emma, or to make peace with her death. My loss filled space and time. Sadness and grief may be with me until I go to heaven, but peace still exists in my heart.

No friend or counselor can change my reality, or take away the void where Emma should be. She is missing like an empty spot from a lost piece of a completed puzzle. My faith assures me she is out there waiting, but I can't reach her and fill in the empty gap.

I don't suppose I will, or should, ever be without thoughts of her. I've come to peace with accepting Emma's disease and death, but accepting the void of her being absent is a mountain I may never tackle. To me, it is sad knowing life must go on without her, but I find God's truth within the sadness.

God never promised happiness, but He has promised joy. Happiness is dependent on circumstances; joy is permanent. "These things I have spoken to you, that *my joy* may be in you, and that your joy may be full" (John 15:11 ESV). "You have sorrow now, but I will see you again, and your hearts will rejoice, and no one will take your joy from you" (John 16:22 ESV). Not even death can take away the joy in my heart, for it is God's joy that is living in me.

I find joy in Jesus, but I will never be completely happy here on earth. My awareness doesn't mean I am unhappy, or depressed. It is simply my reality now. My awareness of life won't keep me from fighting for other children and families who are journeying through the same darkness. It won't keep me from finding laughter in the moments. Truly, God wants us to keep laughing, to continue learning from Emma's life, and to find God's mercy intertwined within pain.

Joy and suffering exists together in this life. Jesus walked to the cross with sadness and pain. He knew what was to happen, yet he had joy knowing what He was about to accomplish.

Truth has taught me many things. I've learned I can find peace in pain, and that the Lord is always present through struggles. I thank God for my pain, and for my happiness. I thank God for my Emma.

In My Dreams

chapter thirteen

*"I lie down and sleep; I wake again,
because the Lord sustains me."* Psalm 3:5

Sleep is a place for wrestling within my psyche. For a long time, my sleep was filled with pain, flashing images of death, tears, and a longing to hold my Emma. There was so much turmoil to reconcile in my mind. My body worked to repair and to heal itself from the traumatic loss. My mind tried to make sense of it all.

Nightmarish dreams of the child who was once alive awoke me again. I pulled myself out of bed to keep the demons from tormenting me. No need to continue trying to sleep when all I saw was my daughter's cold body in front of me.

Sleep was difficult as my brain tried to process Emma's life and death. The nightmares continued for months after she passed away. Her sounds still filled my mind. In my sleep, I could hear her coughing, always a prelude to vomiting. I could hear her oxygen tank humming, and her feeding pump clicking.

Sometimes, I wondered if I was going crazy. The sounds were so very real, so vivid. My body was still on high alert for her sounds, listening for the cue to jump out of bed and run to her room when she needed help.

But the sounds I heard in my dreams were not real. She was not in the other room. Our house became oddly quiet after Emma left.

"How can this be? Emma was so quiet. She didn't make much noise. Why does silence constantly bear down on me, reminding me that she is not here?" I silently questioned.

I missed her before she ever left, but now that she was gone, grief plummeted me like the ocean's tempest—in heartbreaking waves. Sometimes they were small waves. Other times, they were hurricane-sized storm surges that wreaked havoc on my emotional state and threatened to drown me in the dark sea of grief. I found myself gasping for air in grief's surf and onslaught. I had to learn to tread water, to live while breathing in death. Death stole a level of innocence about life from me.

Tears came daily. I felt anger toward the deadly disease which took her from me. I wished Emma would just come back. The ticking clocks of time infuriated me when I thought of how much time had passed since I held my daughter. Time passed so quickly.

The reality of a terminal disease is watching someone you love die. Once they are gone, you experience mixed emotions. On one hand, you know they are finally whole and completely at peace. On the other hand, you live with the reality that they are gone. You miss them and want to hold them again. Grief is both an emotional and a physical state of awareness.

My faith needs assurance, subtle reminders when I feel weak. Blessings, gentle whisperings of faith, came when I need them most. Through every moment, God taught me lessons about appreciating life and our time together here on earth:

- Tell your children and family you love them every day.
- Do not hold grudges; instead, hold one another.
- Existing is not good enough.
- There is life after death.

Chapter 13 *In My Dreams*

Months after Emma's death, a blessing came one dawn as light began to fill the bedroom. I was in that silent cusp of awareness between wake and sleep. I felt Eli stop by my bedside, sit for a moment, put his hand on my back and whisper quiet words in my ear.

"I love you. I am always with you." Then he left.

Warmth, comfort, and peace spread throughout my body. It was odd, though, because Eli never tells me goodbye in the morning.

I heard a door open and shut somewhere downstairs. I opened my eyes, fully awake now. I looked over and found Eli still lying in bed asleep. He hadn't whispered those words. I knew it was the Lord.

"Thank You, Lord, for casting tiny ripples into my pool of faith."

God's light was my beacon. He guided me to the safety of His presence. I stayed in His Word, as much as I could, filling my mind with hope. I relied on God's truth and His promise of peace, even when I had no idea how to make peace arise in my heart.

Before Emma passed into the next life, I experienced anticipatory grief. I knew the reality of what was coming, and I tried to prepare myself as much as possible. I searched for the help and support I would need to make it through. Now I understand there is no preparation for grief.

There is no way to prepare for the impending death of a loved one. All we can do is have a strong support system and pray, pray, pray.

I prayed for comfort, for solace.

I prayed for strength to fully and completely experience the ocean waves of grief.

I prayed God would have mercy on me when the time came to rise from the turbulent ocean surf.

My healing could not happen soon enough for me, but the journey forced me to work slowly through the pain. When I felt particularly down, I would sit quietly and think of her, my "Little Bit." I scoured through her pictures over and over again. I wanted to erase the last image of her that was burned into my mind's camera lens.

I prayed for peace and comfort, and it often came while I looked at photos of me with Emma. I kept myself surrounded by pictures of Emma, mostly from my special time, before she began declining when all of our children together.

She was almost two. She had a head full of curly, red hair. She always wanted to be in my arms, and I adored her. She loved me, but I loved her with a passion from the heart of God.

Looking at pictures of us together and allowing myself to smile resulted in joy and pride slowly beginning to awaken within me. The pictures reminded me of the truth; my love for Emma was alive. She was alive within me.

"Thank you, Lord, for giving wonderful Emma to me for a short while. She led me to desire to learn more about You and the promise we all have if we accept Your truth. I will see her again. Thank you, Lord, for making me Emma's mother."

I began filtering out the raw, painful images that repeated through my mind. I prayed for peaceful images to replace the dark images. Every time my mind ventured to one of the many dark images of Emma dying, I learned to immediately replace the image with a happy, peaceful memory of her instead.

It was an exercise of faith and belief that, someday, peace would overwhelm the pain. And it did.

I began to dream of Emma with vivid clarity. She talked and squealed with delight in my dreams. She would yell, "One! Two! Three!" The way I would do with Paige as we played together. As I slept, Emma would talk to me the way Paige did. In my dreams, all my children played and talked together.

Chapter 13 *In My Dreams*

"Perhaps Emma has always been present," I thought one day. "She is here laughing and squealing with Paige and Peyton, but her sound comes in tiny whispers, inaudible to our human ears. Her laughter is like wind flowing over us. It's separate and from another world, but always present and blending softly into our lives. Emma's essence is somehow becoming a living part of us."

I have come to realize that though the pain of grief may eventually heal, the scar will always be present. I will always miss Emma and long to hold her. I will always feel sad about not having her here with me, but I have an assurance that joy will fully come again.

My soul has ached. It will never fully heal on this earth, but the demons in my dreams have gone away. The sound of her laughter rings in my ears, instead of the sounds of coughing. I hold onto Emma's laughter, which is alive in my dreams. I chose to believe she lives in the full light of Heaven, and I will see her again.

Define Normal

chapter fourteen

Normal: "standard, original, exact, typical"

"It is no longer I who live, but Christ who lives in me, and the life I now life in the flesh, I live by faith in the Son of God, who loved me and gave himself to me." Galations 2:20

The grief journey is a tough one, and the stress weighs heavily on a family. After burying a child, each family takes a different path to move forward. You have to decide how you chose to live the rest of your life after your child dies. None of us choose to be bereaved parents, but afterward, we do have a choice in how we live and move forward.

Adjusting to a "normal" family life with two typical children, meant embarking on yet another journey. The new, more "normal" life was unknown, foreign, and frightening at times. The funny thing is, I had always thought we were a "normal" family with Emma! Because I thought we were normal, we made abnormal seem easy. To the outside world, we were interesting and inspiring. To us, we were simply living everyday life.

Four months after Emma's death, Eli and I began chiseling out a whole new form of discipline, rules, and precedents for our family. Part of our new traditions included ways we would remember Emma. We keep her memory alive and woven securely into the fabric of our family.

Eli and I have not "lost" a child; we still have three. We talk about her. We leave her pictures and favorite things throughout our home. Her blanket and pillow grace our bedroom. We remind Peyton and

Paige that Emma will always be their sister. Her short presence in our lives has eternally impacted our family.

On her birthday we have a small party and take balloons to her grave. We decorated our home in butterfly garlands, and set out little reminders of her. Peyton and Paige would be excited because my mom would bring them presents on Emma's birthday.

On Emma's fifth birthday, our second one without her, I kept wondering if it was appropriate to continue having birthday parties for her. I then remembered rules for "appropriateness" were thrown out the window long ago. We must do what feels right for our family, and it feels right to celebrate the birth of our daughter every July 6th.

We celebrate her entering this world, and the three years, ten months, and sixteen days we had her on earth. We always want Peyton and Paige to smile on July 6th, and remember their very special sister. We want them to feel free to ask questions, laugh, giggle, and look at photos.

A few months after Emma died, I walked into the living room, glanced at her picture and thought to myself, *"It was a simpler time when she was here."* Along with adjusting to our new family, I was trying to discover where my psychological-identity-peg fit into life.

I was a mother to three children, but I had become so enmeshed in Emma's care that my identity was "Mommy to Emma, the child with Cockayne Syndrome, a terminal illness."

Emma held up part of my internal psychological structure. My identity as a mom to Emma defined the "me" I presented to the world and the "me" I perceived myself to be. God wasn't even a part of how I defined myself.

My identity died when my daughter died. I not only had to learn my new family; I had to find the new me. My family needed me, but I had to move through grief to be there for them. As a mother, I wanted

CHAPTER 14 *Define Normal*

to heal from losing Emma, so I could be a better parent for all of my precious children.

I prayed that each of my kids would feel special, unique and loved in their own beautiful, and individual ways. Even in grief, I still spent time with my other children and reveled in the new things they did each day. I still laughed and enjoyed my husband. God's love surrounded me, and I trusted His plan, but an emptiness remained in my heart.

Through time, I'm learning new things about myself I never knew. The depth of my character is found in the lines across my forehead. Deep truth is shadowed in my eyes.

For so long I have grieved, with every fiber of my being, over the death of my daughter. Now, as I look at myself in the mirror, I struggle to understand the person I have become. As I peer at my aging countenance, I am aware of how pain can live, breathe, and over time, transform itself into strength. My new strength has become the foundation for the rest of my life. It gives me a new identity—an identity which recognizes I am so broken I can't fix myself. I recognize how much I need the man called Jesus to intervene.

With Emma gone, I had more freedom in my daily routine. That meant there were huge blocks of time when I would have absolutely nothing to do. Emma wasn't there. There was no one to take care of when Peyton and Paige were in school.

All laundry was done, and the house was clean. Recipes were alphabetized. Dinner no longer consisted of frantically throwing together something semi-edible, turning off smoke alarms, and making the strawberry shortcake into dinner instead of dessert.

My life wasn't chaotic anymore, and I wasn't sure how to cope. I hated to be alone. I needed to keep busy. Why couldn't I just be still?

While Emma was alive, I survived on little sleep. My mind stayed in overdrive keeping up with doctors, medicines, therapies, and comfort measures. I never stopped to breathe. I balanced perilously on the edge of sanity and rarely had time to stop and absorb the monumental whirlwind that was our daily life.

I didn't allow pity, whining, or feeling sorry for our family. I stormed forward with full force ahead, simultaneously taking care of three children, one dog (who was epileptic), one cat (who growled and hissed at anyone human), and a husband who worked his heart out to provide for our family.

I tried to be like the mom on the Kool-Aid commercials I had watched as a kid growing up in the 80's. I was striving to read to, play with, educate, and help my kids meet milestones, all the while being "fun" as I was cleaning up throw-up, washing two, or sometimes three, loads of Emma's clothes and bedding a day, and managing g-tube feedings, oxygen tanks, and twelve medications, all in my head.

I never had time for play dates, lunch dates, cupcakes, park time or any time to be by myself. If you had asked me before Emma died what I did well, the only answer I would have been able to muster with clarity was, "I take very good care of my Emma."

Before, I had been hard on myself when I compared my life to the other moms. Now that I had more time on my hands, I would find myself saying, "Oh! This is how those other moms had time to learn how to cook, and sew, and join a club, go to the park, and do crafts with their kids."

Those moms had kids that could feed themselves, play alone for periods of time, and go to sleep at night.

Those moms were not physically and emotionally drained from dealing with the thought of their child having a terminal illness.

And now *I* was one of *those moms*.

We Give Thanks

chapter fifteen

"But for us, the road unfurls itself, we don't stop walking, we know there is far to go." —Denise Levertov

The morning after Thanksgiving, just six months after Emma died, I awoke with the thought, *"I made it through the first Thanksgiving without her."*

On our first Thanksgiving without Emma, Eli and I decided to have a quiet dinner with just us and the kids. We spent the morning cooking and had a mostly peaceful meal, with the exception of Paige, who refused to sit in her chair. Instead, she perched on daddy's lap as she shoved macaroni and cheese, lima beans, and "choc milk" into her mouth.

Sometime in the late afternoon, we felt ready to be around hordes of family, so we headed down to Eli's parent's house. It was a large gathering of grandparents, two generations of cousins, Eli's favorite aunt and uncle, random friends and boyfriends, and one tiny dog whose response to the chaos was to shake uncontrollably. They all greeted us.

It was loud. There was wine. There was laughter. There were small children fighting over refrigerator magnets and little people toys scattered across the room.

But there was no Emma.

Her pictures adorned her grandparent's home, and her sunny smile reminded us she is always with us in our memories. We laughed, visited with family, and let our kids be kids, but felt Emma's missing presence.

I remembered our last Thanksgiving with Emma. She looked like a tiny Rainbow Bright doll wearing red fleece pants and colorful striped shirt. I topped off the outfit with a small red fleece jacket. She glared at me as I dressed her that day. She looked at Eli as if to say, "Help me out over here!"

He said, "I know, Emma. Mommy has you dressed in hot clothes and looking like a rainbow."

Emma sighed. But she was so cute.

Her tiny image would not show up in the family photos ever again, and for some reason, I refused to have my own picture taken. I didn't want to be in any pictures without Emma. At the time, I was still unable to emotionally decipher why I refused to be in pictures.

On that Thanksgiving Day, I absorbed the grins of my kids as they devoured chocolate pie with cherries. I realized that this first holiday, on the heels of the six-month anniversary of Emma leaving, stood as a hallmark summit in my journey. It marked the beginning of the second half of the first year without Emma.

Six months had passed since Emma left the earth. We had made it through her fourth birthday without her, through July 4th, Peyton starting kindergarten and learning to read, Halloween, Paige's second birthday, and now Thanksgiving.

As the second half of the first year faded from one month to the next, I continued to miss Emma. There were weeks where I was trapped in wells of darkness, but I emerged from each low with insight into the person I was becoming.

I always knew I was meant to be a mother, but now I was learning that God delights in me as His daughter. I realized the God I had

CHAPTER 15 *We Give Thanks*

prayed to for hope, the God I had prayed to for peace, was real. And He alone could change my life.

Seven Months

On the seventh month anniversary of Emma leaving us, just a few days before Christmas, Peyton came to me and asked, "Mommy, is Emma really never coming back?"

"No, Buggy, she is not," I replied. He held onto me for a very long time, sobbing.

Peyton was six, and the reality that death is permanent was sinking into his developing mind. Later on, during the day, he put on a puppet show for Paige and me. One of the ducks in the show died, but his duck friend missed him so much that God brought the dead duck back to life.

My son has always been an extremely bright, compassionate, little boy, filled with boisterous boy-energy. When he was younger, I would sometimes become frustrated with his hyperactive tendencies and headstrong nature, but on this day, sadness crept into my heart as the pain he was obviously feeling seeped out into the pretend world of his puppet show.

We had to be gentler with him and patient, to tread lightly on his young psyche. It is easy to become wrapped up in our adult problems, and not realize that negative behavior is sometimes the language our children's grief speaks. We must hold onto their gentle, sweet spirits as we traverse our grief.

On a December day, the first December after Emma left, I propelled the kids out of the house, and we went to the Dollar Store to buy Christmas gifts for Daddy. Afterward, we went to deliver Christmas cards to our friends at Hospice Family Cares, the hospice that had cared for Emma before she died.

It was wonderful to see Emma's nurses, social worker, and therapist again. Seven months after Emma left us, I was able to wrap my arms around those beautiful women from hospice and say thank you

Paige went right to Jan, Emma's hospice nurse. Jan said she missed seeing Paige at the front door when she would walk up to our home. We laughed about how Paige would try to eat her stethoscope.

Our first Christmas without Emma came too soon. I didn't know what the day would bring, but I knew we would not take the holiday for granted—as if we could take anything for granted anymore. We laughed at Peyton and Paige. We shared in their joy and glee as they feasted their eyes upon their gifts. We took the time to talk about Christ being the true meaning of Christmas, and we spent time thinking about Emma.

On the afternoon of the first Christmas without Emma, our family released a balloon shaped like a butterfly into the air with a note Peyton had written and attached to the string. As we watched the balloon soar into the sky, it veered off into a tree and became stuck. As we all stood there staring at the stuck butterfly balloon, we began to laugh. And somehow, it was okay. We were all laughing together, and we knew Emma was laughing with us.

Countdown

The first New Years Day without Emma passed quickly. Spring came and I found myself at April 22, 2006—thirty days away from the one-year anniversary of Emma's death. Grief was a bear for nearly a year. I had fear about what the thirty-day countdown would hold for me emotionally. How torn by the beast called grief would I become?

Chapter 15 — We Give Thanks

What depths would my soul be driven to as I re-lived the last month of Emma's life? It was intensely excruciating.

Over the previous eleven months, I had watched my grief evolve. As my layers unraveled, I never knew who I would be from one day to the next. In the beginning, I was deeply fragile and utterly exposed—as if I were naked to the world.

The words "Emma is dead" reverberated in my head and her death infiltrated all aspects of my life. I was afraid to be alone in the house. I had absolutely no patience for the tantrums of my other children. I sobbed with such raw emotion and force, I felt my insides may explode.

Then, nearly one year later, I found myself still wounded, but slowly making progress. I was beginning to replace the dreadful moments of her life—the memories which resembled nightmares—with her smiles, her laughter, and her gentle spirit. All that remained was an aching, dull void as I missed seeing her, hearing her, and holding her.

Powerful nightmares haunted my mind as the one-year anniversary loomed. Tears still come and they always will. I've learned when to mention her and when to keep quiet. And finally, I've settled into this new, different life without her. I've learned to go on with life and not feel guilty about laughing, enjoying life, or looking forward to the future.

One Year

May 22, 2006 was the one-year anniversary of Emma's death. I remembered her life by pouring my emotion onto paper. I wrote about the day she was born, and about the day she died.

My Journey with *Emma*

A bursting summer's sun began to light a new day. Emma was born into this world against a backdrop of mountains and a sky radiant with deep pink and indigo hues. We were introduced to her fiery spirit and catapulted into life with a most amazing child. On that sultry summer day, we became trapped in time, caught in rapture as we inhaled joy and absorbed her radiance.

Nearly four years later, butterflies danced through the landscape and flower petals were in full bloom. Our tiny, exquisite Emma, so filled with light, exhaled her last breath and took flight from this world. Her scent, laugh, and delicate imprint will stay on our soul forever.

Emma. Her name meant "the one who heals." It was a tantalizing notion because during her days on earth she seemed so in need of repair, her tiny body refused to adhere to the rules of a healthy childhood. In the wake of her earthly death, the truth came and shone its grace all around. She was not to *be healed*; it was Emma's presence in our lives that healed *us*.

One year after her death, we gingerly stepped through a doorway, the threshold to the rest of the journey. It was filled with uncertainty, but I could see we were kicking at the darkness, and the future was bleeding light.

Light comes. It is the subtle, gentle caress of awareness that Emma's spirit was shaped and filled by God's grace. The feelings of contentment and fulfillment I had when I held her was God infusing Himself into my life through her.

I bask in truth while reflecting on her life, and her amazing journey. Emma was beautifully and wonderfully made. Her genetic fabric was carefully chosen well before she began her life on earth. God placed her into our family where she would be lovingly cared for.

Her syndrome did not debilitate our family, but instead it empowered us. We continue to be amazed by her work here on earth.

CHAPTER 15 *We Give Thanks*

Our family now travels on life's journey without Emma's physical presence, but we feel her spirit with us. Her melodic laughter silently resounds around us.

Thank you, Emma, for the love you gave us, and the lessons you taught us. You blessed each person who met and beheld you. It was never a sacrifice to give all to you, and to absorb all you had to give back. We know why you came, and we are humbled to have been a part of your life.

Too Much Reality

chapter sixteen

"Weep with them that weep." Romans 12:15

My college-aged babysitter presented a speech on Cockayne Syndrome to her class. Afterward, she relayed the class reaction to me. Other students were stunned, in disbelief, and had extreme sadness. One fellow classmate said to her, "I have children and I don't want to think about this sort of thing. This is not something I want to worry with." Another said, "This is too sad. Isn't the mom sad all the time?"

"I am so sorry," I said to my babysitter. "Their reactions are normal though. Most people don't want reality poking into their internal bubble of safety." Having reality careen head-on collision-style into their existence causes defense mechanisms to pop-up.

At one time in my life, I had those same thoughts of denial. I didn't want to acknowledge the harsh possibilities of life. Before Emma, I expected to only have normal problems in life. I thought I was entitled to a fairytale existence. I thought families of mentally and physically challenged children were to be pitied.

Now, I understand truth and see honor in the challenge, the gift from God, of having a special child. Wearing my experience like a badge of courage, I walk through life proud of my child who was born with special needs. I do not care about offending people anymore.

I don't worry about making them uncomfortable by mentioning terminal illness, my sweet daughter Emma, or Cockayne Syndrome.

Knowing When to Speak Up and When to Shut Up

It was the winter festival at Peyton's school. He was in first grade. It was about a year and a half after Emma's death. The school gym was filled with giant inflatable slides. Cotton candy, popcorn and sweets were available galore, and kids were high on sugar.

Children ran all over the place. Volunteer parents were in charge of the various activities. I was the homeroom mom for Peyton's first grade class, so I was in charge of one of the giant bouncy slides. Arriving right on time to relive the previous shift, I met the mom in charge and introduced myself. She had a child in Peyton's class and said hello. Then she proceeded to ask how many children I had. Oh, how I despised that innocent question. I couldn't help it. I just didn't know how to answer it. Did I say two? Three? Two and explain? Three and explain? Lie and say, None! I'm just the aunt!?

Instead, I didn't say anything. I just smiled and nodded toward Peyton and Paige who were standing nearby. I just hoped she did not ask more questions. She looked at my kids and said, "Oh, just two? You must have it easy then. I have *four* kids."

She emphasized the word four, drawling it out as she said the word, "fourrrrrr." Bewildered, I stood there in silence for a few moments as I processed her comment. EASY?

My head filled with thoughts of another time in my life, of having three children. One hooked to feeding pumps and oxygen. One

Chapter 16 — Too Much Reality

desperately needing attention. One learning to walk as she tip-toed over oxygen tank tubing. One dying in my arms.

Easy was not a word I would have used to describe life. Then I realized the other mom must have meant I had it easy because we only had two children.

In the nearly two years since Emma's death, I had learned there was a fine line between mentioning Emma and keeping quiet about her. I stayed silent for a moment, pondering on whether this was a time to keep quiet, but I innately knew it was a time to mention Emma.

After a few moments which seemed like eternity, I replied, "Well, I do have three children. But my daughter Emma died a year and a half ago. Actually, it seemed easier when there were three in our home."

Her expression was shocked and baffled, but she managed to sputter, "Easier, really?"

No more words were spoken between that woman and myself. There were only polite smiles. She didn't say "hello" when we passed one another at school functions. She made a quick beeline for the nearest exit when she saw me. But she was the one who asked how many children I had . . .

Did I have to mention Emma? No. Did I need to? Yes.

Sometimes people need a glimpse into another reality that is not their own. I did not mention Emma in order to offend, or frighten that woman. I mentioned Emma because it was necessary to offer a glimpse into my reality. I needed to let the woman know that we all have struggles, and that you can't know or judge what someone is walking in simply by what you perceive to be their life.

There is a quote by Shannon L. Alder that I can't get away from. It is long, but it perfectly describes the importance of breaking silence. It reads:

Silence never healed the lonely. Silence never comforted the broken hearted. Silence never saved a life. Silence never won an argument with kindness. Silence never healed the poor. Silence never learned compassion. Silence never saw the pain in another. Silence never asked for forgiveness. Silence never felt remorse. Silence never felt empathy. Silence never grew up. Silence never listened to promptings. Silence never resolved a problem. Silence never had closure. Silence never had a conscience. Silence never developed integrity. Silence never knew manners. Silence never learned respect. Silence never matured. Silence never understood that the Bible and its stories was God's way of saying, 'Stop being silent and start healing one another.' Silence never realized that Christ was an activist for communication.

No Whining

While Emma was alive, I placed a handmade sign with the words "NO WHINING!" on the front door. I put it there to remind my four-year-old son he was not allowed to whine downstairs. I hung up another sign in his room that said, "WHINING ALLOWED!" Peyton eventually learned the lesson in positivity, but I didn't remove the sign on our front door. It was a lesson I continued to teach to Paige.

I haven't mentioned it before, but a newspaper reporter followed our family for six months prior to Emma's death in order to write a story on Emma's journey. One day, he noticed the sign and asked about it. I told him the truth. I made that sign out of desperation in trying to deal with a raving-mad four-year-old.

Over time, our whole family adopted the "no whining" policy. It has become our mantra. We were not going to whine about what we

CHAPTER 16 *Too Much Reality*

faced and dealt with in life. We were going to absorb it, learn from it, teach others, and thank God for whatever He placed before us.

NO WHINING! The reporter wrote about that handmade sign in the newspaper when he described our family. Several years after I taped the NO WHINING sign up, it was time to take it down. Two years after Emma died, I placed the sign into a box and carted it off to the new home we moved into. The sign took residence in our new house and many years later, it still remains hanging on the front door.

At first, it did not seem possible we could ever call another house "home." How could it be home without memories of Emma living within the walls? But as we settled into our new house, our family discovered that Emma is always with us. Her memory is not within a house; it is in each of us. We find her in the shine which lights up Peyton's face as he tells funny stories about her. Emma is with us as we meet other children with Cockayne Syndrome and take them into our arms without hesitation or fear. Her lingering laughter still fills our new home from within our memories.

The two-year anniversary of Emma going to heaven approached in a different way than the first year did. By the second year, the beast I have always called grief relinquished much of its power over me. Dread, which was so overwhelming as the one-year anniversary approached, didn't not haunt my mind the second year, nor any of the years following.

I have come to realize the anniversary of her death, and the calendar of time passing does not mean my grief should be "all done," "better," or "over." Years gone by will not erase her memory. Instead, I am overcome with revelation. There is a dual meaning found in a person's death date. For those left behind, the date signifies an ending. We feel sorrow as we remember that last day, and the last breath Emma took.

But May 22, 2005, means something totally different for Emma than it does for us. That day marks her homecoming, the glorious day she returned to the One who sent her. It was her first day in a perfect body, free from pain.

Long ago, our pastor taught us to be wary of "signs" or "symbols," and not to place our faith in coincidences, but I do believe Emma's birthdate was significant. Emma was born on July 6, 2001. July is the seventh month in the year. The number seven is significant in the Bible. Her birthday was 07/06/01. When I add the "6," plus the "01," of her birthdate, I get "7."

In the Bible, the number seven represents completion. Emma's life was completed here on earth. She did all she was supposed to do, and then she left.

The day she died, May 22, 2005, Jesus welcomed her home. Welcome home, little girl. May you soar on wings far beyond our touch.

Lessons from my Children

chapter seventeen

"To start from the self and try to understand all things is delusion. To let the self be awakened by all things is enlightenment." —Dogen

I am here for my children who are still walking with me on earth. They need me to be their mother, and fully involved with their lives. But there is a part of me doesn't allow me to be wholly theirs. The adrenaline I lived on during Emma's life has drained out. How did I function when Emma was here? It is a struggle to find focus now, to decipher and muddle through the lessons of Emma's short life, but God has a way of capturing my attention.

When Peyton was around six-years-old he came to me one night before bedtime. He told me a story of Jesus, and linked the story to Emma. Peyton described how Jesus came to complete a job on earth, and when he did what God wanted him to do, Jesus left. Peyton said God had an important job for Emma too. Her job was to help everyone know how much God loves them, and Emma didn't have to live very long to do what God wanted her to do.

Peyton knows and accepts God's truth. He tells me he believes. I feel both tremendous pride and a humble spirit when I think about him. This child, to whom I have given birth, is amazing. It seems he knows more than I do about life. He is so accepting. As his parents, I don't feel we deserve him. He carries so much in his heart, a reality completely different from my own. He had to say goodbye to a little sister.

Just like God had a job for Emma, God has a job for Peyton. God placed Peyton into our family to teach us wisdom and faith. He is also here to learn from our family. Peyton, he is a wonder.

Paige doesn't remember her big sister very much, but because of Emma's life, Paige is a compassionate child who is learning to understand the power of God's love. She knows that while life is not always easy, God is always good. Recently, I pulled out Emma's baby book. Stuck in between the pages was a ziplock baggie with curls of Emma's hair.

I gasped and said, "Her hair!"

Paige was sitting next to me, and her eyes widened in surprise. I carefully took out Emma's curl of hair and held it up. We sat there mesmerized as we both slowly came to the realization that Paige's hair is now the exact same shade of strawberry blonde as Emma's once was. It was a reminder to me that God is in every detail. While Paige doesn't remember her sister as much as she would like, to see this tangible bit of evidence of a sister who was so very real and similar to her, was a gift from God.

I know our children will be okay. They have had the freedom to grieve, ask questions, express their feelings, and embrace heartache alongside laughter. They have had to experience very difficult things at young ages, but they are filled with insight, compassion, and a level of awareness that is amazing.

I teach my children to strive for happiness, but not to expect it to come easily all of the time. Happiness is what you make out of life. My life is full of happiness. I find it in the soulful faces of my children as they seek my approval. I find it in their giggles as we envelop ourselves in make-believe play. I find it in the joy I see on my husband's face when

CHAPTER 17 *Lessons from my Children*

he walks in the door and our children look at him with adoration and hurl themselves onto him for hugs.

I lived most of my life before Emma entangled in a façade. I lived knowing the façade existed, but I fought against the fear I had of revealing my truth—my vulnerability—as I tried to meet the expectations of other people and their social standards. In the first holidays after Emma's death, some family members didn't approve of Eli and I keeping holidays low key and at home with just Peyton and Paige. They said we were isolating them and they didn't agree with how we chose to celebrate.

Over the years, we have learned not to conform to other's beliefs about how we should be acting or what we should be doing in the wake of Emma's death. We will celebrate her birthday and won't be afraid to share her story, her pictures or our journey. As a proud mama, I will continue to mention her name and feel tremendous pride in having the honor of being her parent. I'll stay true to my beliefs as I teach my children about life and death. I am free from the society's cage of "right, appropriate, and necessary."

Emma, Peyton, and Paige sharing a hug

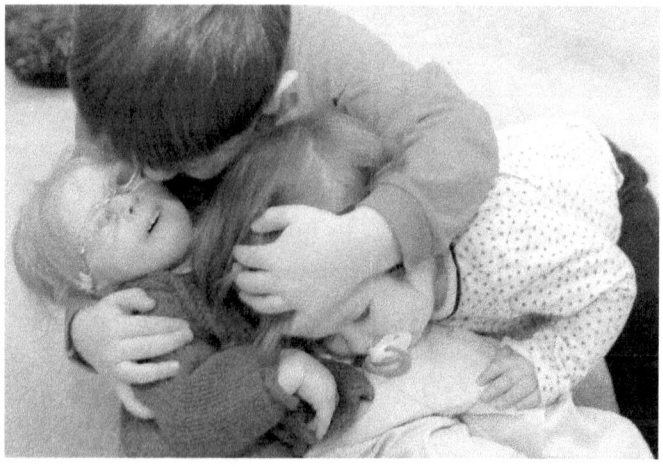

Be Still and Know

chapter eighteen

"Shame says that because I am flawed, I am unacceptable. Grace says though I am flawed, I am cherished." —Unknown

Peace is unbound to material belongings. It is the feeling of being complete with absolutely nothing but love from God, your family, and closest friends. Peace comes from having the Spirit of God live inside of you, filling you up. Peace exists without a heartbeat, and beats stronger than any life force. I had to find that peace—that joy—and it took time.

Two years after Emma's death, I faced my self-façade once again. For weeks I had been feeling the days bear down on me. I felt sluggish, vulnerable, and trapped in invisible quicksand. Each time I would attempt to take a step forward, I sunk further into the immobilizing gunk that kept me from finding truth. Suspended in a state of deep reflection, I was unable to process my thoughts, motivate myself to complete tasks, return calls, or even laugh. I seldom even prayed while in those trenches. Despite all of that, I began to feel an overwhelming need to spend time strengthening and reconnecting my bond with God.

Humbled by my earthly incapability, I bowed down in prayer. Screaming out in sheer frustration, I call on a Power beyond myself to calm my heart. Finally, I find a voice resonating above all the noise.

"Be still and know I am God."

Calm came with that voice, and I knew I could trust Him. His voice was unspoken, but so urgent, and clear in my head.

"Be still and know I am God. Just be."

Once again, I began to feel His soft gentle voice speaking to me. I felt Him slowly pull me out of the quicksand. As I inhaled deeply, I felt my deflated form filling with life again. With that prayer, I started living in the place and time of the moment, accepting each thing the Lord gives me. I'm absorbing it all, and I know the stage I am in now is exactly where God wants me to be.

After being housed in its cocoon, the butterfly senses it is time to emerge. Finally, it breaks free and is able to use its wings to soar. The butterfly reminds me that Emma's earthly body was only preparation for the soaring freedom and peace she now has.

I could see myself like the butterfly too. I was anxious to break free of the cocoon I was living in for so long. I find freedom in truth, peace in pain, and grace in imperfection.

Time keeps moving ahead, but I am not trying to keep up. I now walk through life in my own time, according to how God directs me. My never ending journey with Emma has taught me that only God knows what is right, appropriate, and necessary for my life.

"I am the vine; you are the branches." John 15:5

One quiet evening as the sun was sinking into the deep blink that is darkness, I sat on our long New Orleans style front porch and became absorbed with an epiphany. Gazing through tree limbs, which stretched far and wide across my view, I watched the sky change as the colors of twilight began to paint the horizon.

A thought grew inside me like wildfire. While gazing at the trees and the brilliant color-filled sky, I understood how strong our God is and how far reaching His love is. He is the vine and we are the

CHAPTER 18 Be Still and Know

branches. Even though the tiniest at the top of the tree seems fragile, it is still connected to the strong, powerful, life-giving force. We are each connected to a powerful force, supporting us and beckoning us to remain close. At times, life consumes us and we become far from Him, but He is always there. We are the branches. He is the vine, our anchor of spiritual strength.

Surrounded by the quiet collapse of daylight, I breathed in the knowledge of how easy it is to feel separate from the world when going through deeply painful experiences. But God is not of this world. I am reminded that this world will someday fade away. But a spiritual power will always be with us, guiding us toward hope. It is hope, the absolute knowing that I am connected to a powerful God who loves me and Emma, which allows me to have a supernatural solace. It is why when people ask how I am OK, I am able to answer, "Only God."

The calm I now feel about Emma's life and her leaving is as powerful and palpable as the pain I have walked through.

> "It is better to go to the house of mourning than to go to the house of feasting, for this is the end of all mankind, and the living will lay it to heart." Ecclesiastes 7:2

I always struggled with why the Bible said it was better to go into a house of mourning than a house of feasting, until one Sunday when our pastor's message centered on Ecclesiastes 7:2.

In my sense of understanding, of Solomon's writings in Ecclesiastes paints the "house of feasting" as a celebration where we are focused on fun, food, and what we see on the surface. We have a good time at the house of feasting. And why not? After all, isn't that what we are supposed to be doing at a celebration? God wants us to enjoy life.

But Solomon writes that it is better to go into a house of mourning.

We go into a "house of mourning" with the death of loved ones. We mourn with friends, through difficult times, and while serving orphans and widows in their grief. In the house of mourning, we focus on our own mortality. We think about things we have or haven't accomplished, and areas of our life we want to nourish.

We become introspective and forced to face issues that have remained beneath the surface for too long. The house of mourning forces us to think about death, our own death, and the death of our loved ones. By telling us it's better to enter a house of mourning, Solomon wants us to think about God and where we will spend eternity.

A house of mourning is where we are most vulnerable to the truth, because our facades have all fallen away. In the house of mourning, we make decisions which can change our lives. We look inward while walking through a house of mourning.

I've been looking inward for a long time. So long, I often wonder if my inside is actually what everyone sees now. For me, embracing a house of mourning has shown me it's okay to let people see I am imperfect. It's okay for my children and my marriage to be imperfect. It's okay to say I leave food in the fridge until it gets all moldy at times.

I've learned it's okay to be authentic, and to show my flaws because God has covered my flaws with His blood, and His grace. By being open about my brokenness I show how God is healing my heart. By entering a house of mourning, I am growing closer to the heart of God and my own salvation.

Legacy

chapter nineteen

"Hope is grief's best music." —Unknown

As I write, I have struggled to find an endpoint to *My Journey with Emma*. I keep looking for a point of completion, but one more truth I am realizing is **there is no end**. There does not have to be an ending to this story.

Truth forever carves out who I am today and who I will be tomorrow. Truth brings solace, comfort, and peace. Truth finds my identity in Christ. Truth leads me to find happiness in the quietness of my soul. Truth is a personal connection with God.

His love covers everything I do. His love is greater than anything I can imagine here on earth. I don't have to be perfect, or present a façade to the world. Admitting failure, fear, and weakness is exactly where God wants me to be.

God meets me where I am and breaks down the boundaries that surround me. He removed the walls which surrounded the person I was before. He broke through my layers of materialism, until one day I found my inner self in His presence. He blends me together, all of my suffering and joy, to make an imperfect person who is unashamedly covered in grace and forgiveness.

Every day, I face the fact I can't live a perfect life, but every day I experience God's joy. I have always known God created me as a writer.

My Journey with Emma

I never imagined He would use my child to inspire me to write a book of His love.

In 2011, God opened our hearts to love in yet another way—adoption. Adoption is very important to God's heart. We see it all throughout the Bible. We have been blessed beyond measure to bring home our youngest child, through adoption, when she was four-years-old.

Her name is Svetlana Josie (Sveta Josie) and she has enriched our lives by showing us a glimpse of God's heart we never would have known had it not been for adoption. I wrote much of this book before Sveta came into our lives, but God is in her story too.

God led us to Sveta in the fall of 2010 when I learned about a child with Cockayne Syndrome living in an orphanage in Ukraine. I began to advocate for that little girl to have a family and an amazing family adopted her.

God continued to whisper into my heart, "I'm not done." One day, a friend told me about a little girl she had met while adopting her children in Ukraine. The little girl had big blue eyes. Something about the child captured her heart.

My friend put me in contact with a missionary at the orphanage who sent our family a 10-second video of a girl riding around the yard in a little red car. We all hovered around my computer and watched the little girl sing a little song in Russian. Eli and I, along with Peyton and Paige, sat quietly and didn't say a word as we absorbed what we had just taken in. We all knew this child was meant to be in our family and we would travel across the world to a place called Nikolaev, Ukraine, to bring her home.

We began the journey with Sveta in January 2011, and she came home in July 2011. God gave me her middle name as I was looking at a photo of her asking Him, "What is her name?"

CHAPTER 19 *Legacy*

I clearly heard God say, "Josie."

I told Eli. He agreed she looked like a Josie. A few days later, I looked up the meaning of the name Josie. It means "God will multiply." God has certainly multiplied our family through adoption, but He has also multiplied our awareness of His love for the fatherless. It is difficult to describe what God did in our hearts with Sveta and adoption. He showed us love beyond genetics, a deep compassion for the fatherless, and hope in grief. He gave us another child, and we have rejoiced in our Sveta, who we call "little one."

Sveta is compassionate and sweet. God has surrounded her with peace. We are so completely humbled that God has allowed us to be her parents. Peyton and Paige completely accepted Sveta and they were right alongside us as we made the decision to adopt. The bond God has created between Paige and Sveta is beautiful to watch. They are true sisters.

In God's funny way of timing, we took Sveta out of the orphanage late on the evening of July 5th. Her first full day with us was July 6th, 2011—Emma's 10th birthday. His timing wasn't lost on us. I recall laughing and thinking "God gave us our Sveta on Emma's 10th birthday!" He never ceases to amaze me. Miracles still happen, just like this.

Eli and I, along with Sveta and two Ukrainian facilitators, piled into a van the morning of July 6th to make the 6-hour drive to Kiev. As we drove, we hit giant Ukrainian road potholes, causing us to lurch into the ceiling of the car. Eli and I could only laugh as we listened to Sveta yell in Russian to stop the car. We laughed, prayed, and praised God for our child.

God has continued to press upon our heart over children who are hurting and needing families. After international adoption, we felt called to help children in the U.S. through foster care, and possibly adoption once again. We have learned to say "yes" to God and know He doesn't make mistakes. We are learning to live with a servant's heart and show Peyton, Paige, and Sveta what living with a servant's heart looks like. It's saying "yes" to God even when it doesn't make sense.

Our children are growing up. This year, Peyton is 17. Paige is 13, and Sveta is 9. They are thriving and happy. They are avidly involved in hockey, soccer, and musical theater. They bring us joy.

Peyton is working ahead in his classes and is almost finished with high school. He wants to join the military and is exploring different branches. He works on a landscaping crew and is one of the most mature, intelligent, and insightful kids most people meet!

Paige is involved in soccer and has a heart to help anyone in need. She is full of compassion and a deep love for the Lord. I've always said she is pure joy and we should have named her Joy. Truly, our Paige is joy personified.

Sveta, our little one, enjoys expressing herself through musical theater, gymnastics and snuggling on the couch to read with me every day. Sveta is an answered prayer, a little girl God gave us unexpectedly. We are the lucky ones because God made us her parents.

My three children are very close. They pick on one another, fight, forgive, hug, and laugh. God has brought us full circle. I know Emma is smiling upon us and enjoying watching her siblings with joy.

One of the most difficult things a parent who has buried a child faces is the fear that their child will be forgotten. We know the Lord knows our Emma and holds her in His hands, but we want to make sure her legacy lives. Her life and death taught us so much, and leads us to show others there is peace in pain, joy in suffering, and hope for new life—all found in Jesus. We pray God's mercy and overwhelming love will be revealed through Emma's story.

CHAPTER 19 *Legacy*

In the years since Emma passed away, Eli and I created a nonprofit organization called *Circle of Hope* to help the families of children with life threatening illness, as well as families adopting children with special needs. I find joy as I pour myself out and wrap those hurting families up in love. We are honored to walk with these families as they journey down difficult roads of grief and loss. As we meet those families in their pain, Emma's life and legacy come into a full *Circle of Hope*.

There are many families we have been honored to help. These families have needed support through volunteers helping with day-to-day activities with terminally ill children, mothers and fathers who have needed help paying for funeral costs and headstones for their children, and families who just needed an ear to listen as they cried.

Circle of Hope impacts families by encircling them with hope and direct support. *Circle of Hope* has been blessed to exist on donations. All donations go to families who are facing medical bills, funeral costs, adoption fees, and other related needs. We are a volunteer organization, and humbly give back everything we bring in to the families God places in our lives. The very real need for *Circle of Hope* is tremendous and we would love you to join us in helping the families and children we are honored to serve. All proceeds from *My Journey With Emma* go to *Circle of Hope* and the families it serves.

As we remember Emma and her very special purpose here on earth, we look forward to the day we will see her again. Though sometimes it feels we are walking through the desert, we will always keep Emma's memory alive and her legacy an integral part of our family. Year after year, we will celebrate her. We know life on earth is not forever, but love, love never dies.

> "Behold, I am doing a new thing; now it springs forth, do you not perceive it? I will make a way in the wilderness and rivers in the desert." Isaiah 43:19

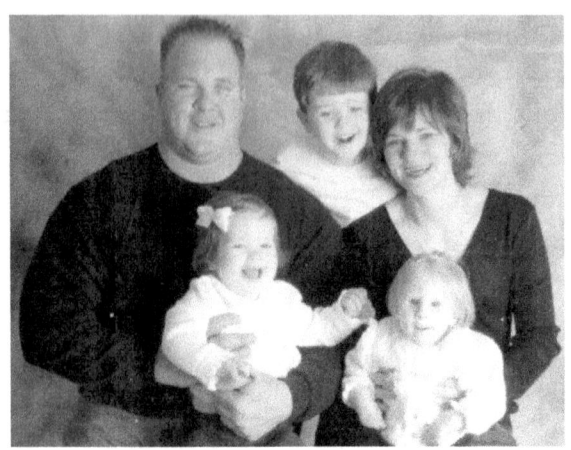

Houser Family, 2005
Eli, Peyton, Kim, Paige, and Emma

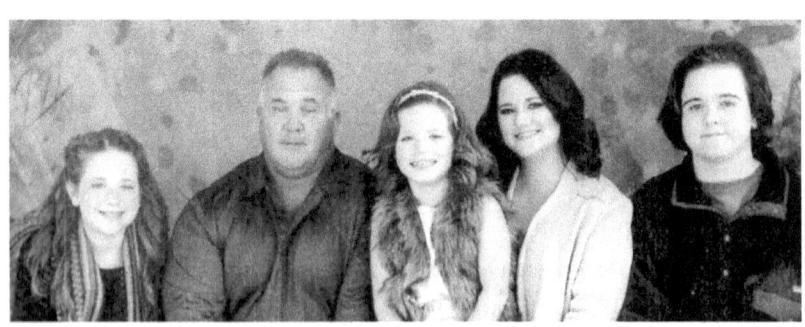

Houser Family, 2016
Paige, Eli, Sveta, Kim, and Peyton

Acknowledgments

My Savior, my Father in Heaven. I humbly wrote these words to bring glory to You, my Redeemer. Thank You for giving Emma to us, for making her our little girl on earth for a short time. Thank You for hope. We know, one beautiful day, we will once again wrap Emma in our arms, as if no time has passed.

My Eli. You are my best friend, the one God chose for me, the one I am humbled to walk this journey of life alongside. You are a devoted father and the one who makes me feel I am the most special person on earth. God brought us together at such very young ages, and I can't imagine life without you. I am so happy to walk life's road with you, through hard times and joyous times. You are the person who loves me most, the person I would choose over, and over again. Thank you for supporting me and telling me to never give up on bringing this story to life.

My precious children, Peyton, Paige and Sveta. You are my laughter, my joy, my pride, the legacy I leave behind. I am so proud of each of you and honored I get to hear each of you call me "Mom." My dear children, you make me smile and make my heart full. Thank you for holding on and staying strong as your mama wrote this book. There were a lot of teary moments. Trust in the Lord, He is the only One who will never let you down.

My Mama and Daddy. You understand me more than I understand myself most of the time and you have loved me with an unconditional love my entire life. You gave me both roots, and wings to fly. I love you both desperately.

My stepmom Laurie. We have a heart connection and a bond of loss. You and Gabe are so dear to me. I know Gabe is with Emma and that brings me great comfort.

My family. Wes, Autumn, Ella, Bailey, Russell, Cecilia, Jed, Sarah, Remy, Matt, Kari, Mable, Leona, my dear uncle Jerry, my aunts Louise and Gale, my cousins Corey, Terri, Darlene and their families. Thank you to the ones who walked through the joy of loving Emma and the pain of saying goodbye to her, and most of all, to each of you, thank you for being a part of our lives.

My friends, Haylee, Ashley, and Katherine. Thank you for your love, your encouragement and always making me laugh, and for putting up with me, I know it's not easy.

My childhood friends, Stacy, Megan, and Wendy. We were new mothers together and you helped me walk through the fire of deep loss. I love each of you so very much.

Gwen. God brought us together as young mothers, he bonded us through our girls. You have been a stronghold of support from the time Emma was a baby. Your friendship is so precious.

The women who helped plan Emma's funeral, Katie, Jennifer, and Patti. You are each a treasure I hold in my heart from a deeply special time, so long ago.

Pastor Keith. You walked with us through the shadow of death and shined truth all the way. Thank you.

Sandra. Thank you for being there that morning and for listening to God, you are engraved on my heart and a part of the story I will never forget.

Rachael, my editor and publisher. You are the last piece to the puzzle of the marvelous plan God had in store for bringing Emma's story to fruition. Thank you for your compassion, your belief in this story, your guidance, your unwavering words of encouragement, your love for the Lord, and for pursuing God's path.

About the Author

Kim Houser

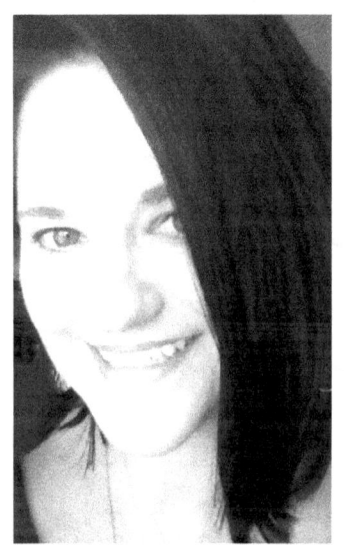

Kim Houser is a self-proclaimed imperfect person, a daughter of the King who relies on His grace every day. She is a passionate advocate for children with special needs, as well as the fatherless and orphans.

She is the co-founder of Circle of Hope, a non- profit organization which provides services and support to families of children with special needs and to families adopting children with special needs.

Through speaking engagements, Kim spreads her passion for adoption, orphan care, and how God's unfailing love can bring hope when all hope seems lost.

Her daughter, Emma, passed away from Cockayne Syndrome at the age of three. Kim's Journey with Emma has been the catalyst for a lifetime dedicated to sharing hope with others.

Kim resides in Alabama with her husband, Eli, and their three children, Peyton, Paige and Sveta.

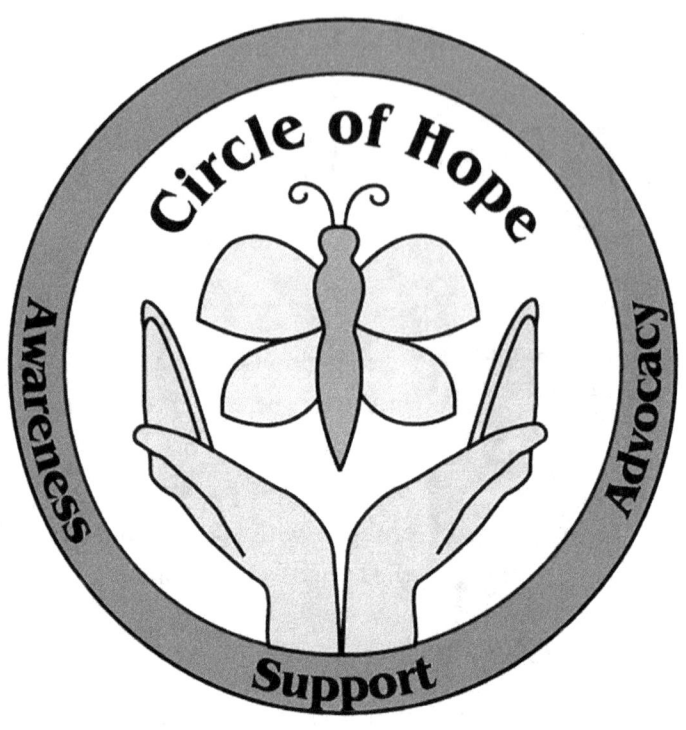

Proceeds from this book go to support Circle of Hope.

Circle of Hope provides support and services to families of children with life threatening and chronic conditions.

In addition, we firmly believe in God's commandment to care for the fatherless and strive to help bring children into forever homes both locally and globally.

You can help by supporting our mission through volunteering, spreading word of our organization to families who may need help, donating and most importantly, through prayer.

circleofhopehuntsville@gmail.com
http://circleofhopehuntsvil.wixsite.com/cohcare

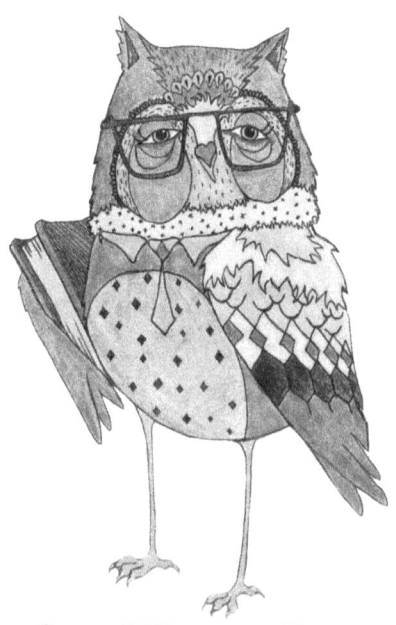

Our Written Lives
book publishing services
www.OurWrittenLives.com

www.ingramcontent.com/pod-product-compliance
Lightning Source LLC
Chambersburg PA
CBHW071740080526
44588CB00013B/2106